An Introduction to Public Health and Epidemiology

An Introduction to Public Health and Epidemiology

Second Edition

Susan Carr, Nigel Unwin and Tanja Pless-Mulloli

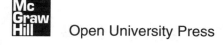

Open University Press

Open University Press
McGraw-Hill Education
McGraw-Hill House
Shoppenhangers Road
Maidenhead
Berkshire
England
SL6 2QL

email: enquiries@openup.co.uk
world wide web: www.openup.co.uk

and
Two Penn Plaza
New York, NY 10121–2289, USA

First edition published 1997
First published 2007

A catalogue record of this book is available from the British Library

ISBN10: 0 335 21624 2 (pb)   0335 21625 0 (hb)
ISBN13: 978 0 335 21624 6 (pb)   978 0 335 21625 3 (hb)

Library of Congress Cataloging-in-Publication Data
CIP data has been applied for

Typeset by RefineCatch Limited, Bungay, Suffolk
Printed in Poland EU by OZGraf S.A.
www.polskabook.pl

The **McGraw·Hill** Companies

To our families.

Contents

Preface

People who practise public health come from many walks of life:

- nurses and doctors running screening programmes;
- local residents campaigning for better housing;
- engineers drilling bore holes to provide clean water for villagers in a developing country;
- politicians introducing legislation to ban cigarette smoking in public places;
- 'pop stars' who speak to school children on the dangers of drug misuse.

These are a few examples. Many people will not identify their activities as 'public health'. What links these and similar activities together is improving the health of populations or communities. Such a broad range of activities illustrates that the factors which influence health are complex and wide-ranging. Any attempt to understand and change them must involve many disciplines, and the study of public health draws on the expertise of people from a variety of backgrounds. Statistics, psychology, sociology, microbiology, politics and management are some of the specialities which contribute to the study of public health. Epidemiology has a central role. It can be defined as the study of the distribution and determinants of health-related states and the application of this study to the control of health problems. Knowing the extent of health problems, who suffers from them and what causes them within a population is the information needed for organized public health groups to address them, as well as the measure of whether the efforts were successful.

The focus of public health is on populations and communities. This is a very different perspective from the day-to-day focus of most health professionals on the health problems of individuals. We hope in this book to introduce students and practitioners of nursing and other health and social care workers to the 'public health perspective', to provide a framework for examining public health issues and to allow the reader to start to place her or his practice within the wider context of health, and determinants of health, of the community in which they work.

This book is a study guide. Our goal is to encourage you to think through, and be critical about, key issues to do with the measurement and improvement of public health and the role in this played by organized health care. The chapters cover topics which we hope will enable this goal to be achieved. There may be other areas you feel we should have covered. We would very much welcome your feedback on the content and any other aspect of this book.

How to use this book

Each chapter has a standard format and is presented in the following way:

- *Questions*: some examples of the kinds of questions the chapter will help you to answer.
- *Outcomes*: what you should be able to do after working through the chapter and the exercises provided.
- *Exercises*: these are presented throughout the chapter. They are there to help you understand key issues. It is therefore important to work through them. You'll be pleased to hear that most of them are very short. There are a few exercises that will involve going away and seeking out other information, but these are identified in the text and are optional. They are there if you wish to develop further your understanding of a particular issue.
- *Summary*: key issues, ideas or concepts from the chapter are identified in summary questions. Spaces are left for your responses for two main reasons: (1) by completing this section you can revise the issues of the chapter and assess for yourself how well you have met the outcomes; (2) you can make your own summary specific to your particular health interests and your branch of health or social care.
- *Public health standards*: at the end of each chapter a table is provided which lists ten public health standards. You are invited to consider which are pertinent to the chapter content, to reflect on your current skills and knowledge, and to develop action plans to address any learning needs.

At the end of the book we have identified some useful references and resources relating to each chapter for further exploration of the chapter subject.

Chapter 1, 'Lessons from the history of public health and epidemiology for the twenty-first century', defines concepts underpinning the evolution of epidemiology and public health thinking. It then places public health successes within a historical context and highlights remaining challenges.

Chapter 2, 'Sources and critical use of health information', provides an overview of the different types of information that are relevant to public health practice. Criteria are suggested by which to assess critically the quality of routinely available health information. The application of these criteria is illustrated by consideration of routinely available information on population size and cause of death. Next, the types of information routinely available on morbidity (episodes of illness) are considered and the concept of the health care iceberg is introduced. Finally, consideration is given to the potential pitfalls when making comparisons between the health of populations in different places or at different times when using routinely collected information.

Chapter 3, 'Measuring the frequency of health problems', starts by illustrating the need for rates to measure the frequency of health problems. Two rates of special importance in epidemiology, incidence and prevalence, are defined and their relationship is discussed. The rest of the chapter uses mortality rates (because these tend to be the most widely used indicators of the 'health' of a population) as an example to illustrate what is meant by crude, specific and standardized rates. Finally, calculation of age-standardized rates by both the direct and indirect methods is illustrated, and the potential shortcomings of both approaches are discussed. Two of the main aims of epidemiology are to identify possible causes of disease and to estimate the potential improvement in a population's health if such causes are removed. Measures of 'relative risk' (and the identification of 'risk' factors) and 'attributable risk' respectively are the main methods by which these aims are met.

Chapter 4, 'Measures of risk', illustrates the meaning of the terms 'hazard' and 'risk' and seeks to encourage a critical approach to their use and interpretation.

Chapter 5, 'Epidemiological study designs', provides an overview of the approaches (study designs) used in epidemiology to measure the extent of a disease or health state in a population and to identify possible causes of a disease or health state. A classification of the different study designs is given and each is described. Emphasis is given to the strengths and weaknesses of the different types of study.

Chapter 6, 'Weighing up the evidence from epidemiological studies', is all about interpreting the results from epidemiology studies. An association between a disease and health state and a possible cause may not be real but owing to 'bias', 'confounding' or 'chance'. These terms are defined and illustrated, and methods for addressing them in the design and analysis of epidemiology studies are discussed. Finally, even if an association is real, it does not necessarily follow that it is 'causal'. What is meant when we describe something as a 'cause' of a disease or health state is discussed and criteria are suggested by which causality can be assessed.

Chapter 7, 'The determinants of health and disease', defines and identifies proximal and distal determinants of disease. The nature of the relationship between poverty and public health is discussed. This is followed by a critical account of the theory of the epidemiological transition. Finally, there is an overview of the demographic characteristics and disease patterns in different parts of the world.

Chapter 8, 'Health promotion', describes the different types of activity which come under the heading of health promotion. Health education is one of the activities coming under the umbrella of health promotion, to which health care workers often contribute. Five different approaches or models of health education are discussed. The reader is encouraged to consider critically where the balance between individual and collective responsibility for health should lie. Issues for consideration in attempting to evaluate health promotion are considered. The reader is encouraged to engage in reflection on their own health promotion practice.

A consideration of the term 'health needs assessment' begs the questions of what is meant by 'health' and what is meant by 'need'? Chapter 9 begins by addressing both these questions. A classification of need is given. Chapter 7 illustrates that determinants of health can be seen to operate on many levels and similarly health needs can be identified on many levels. A particular example of health needs assessment is community health profiling. What is meant by this and how it might be approached is discussed and a framework for considering a community health profile is suggested. Action planning for health is discussed and consideration is given to the contribution of health impact assessment.

Screening individuals to prevent or cure a disease is a deceptively attractive idea. Increasing numbers of health care workers are being asked to undertake screening as part of their day-to-day work. However, a poorly thought out and badly implemented screening programme may be ineffective or, worse still, harmful. Chapter 10, 'Principles of screening', considers the rational criteria for selecting a condition to be targeted in a screening programme. It also considers some of the factors which contribute to the successful implementation of a screening programme.

Chapter 11, 'Changing public health: what impacts on public health practice?', considers how evidence is used to set priorities and to change public health practice. The influence of perception of risk on priority setting is explored. An analysis of the contribution to and impact of a range of stakeholders on the public health endeavour is undertaken. The chapter concludes with a discussion of the importance of, and approaches to, evaluating the impact of public health practice in order to inform future practice.

INTRODUCTION

This book provides an introduction to public health and epidemiology. We hope that by working through all, or sections, of the book the reader will not only increase their knowledge of public health practice but also develop a critical, questioning approach to the application of that knowledge.

Before starting to work on this second edition we asked for feedback from users of the first edition. Based on the feedback received we added two new chapters (1 and 11) and made several other substantial revisions. The first new chapter is on the history of epidemiology and public health, while Chapter 11 considers what actually changes the public health. Chapters 2 and 7 (on information sources and determinants of health respectively) have been largely rewritten. All the chapters have been brought up to date. However, the basic study guide format remains the same. Each chapter begins with a list of questions and learning objectives, uses exercises to help illustrate and develop critical thinking on key points and provides the reader with a framework to write their own summary at the end of the chapter.

Changing and protecting the public health requires a broad range of knowledge and skills. These are summarized in the standards developed in the United Kingdom for specialist public health practitioners (comparable standards exist for other countries). These standards are given below, and they provide a useful checklist for reflecting on your own knowledge and skills. We suggest that you use them as a template to assess your learning needs, process of learning and achievements. They are presented again at the end of each chapter to enable you to reflect on what aspects of these standards that chapter helped you on.

Standards for specialist public health practitioners

1 Surveillance and assessment of the population's health and well-being:

   - health needs assessment;
   - health determinants;
   - health surveillance.

2 Promoting and protecting the population's health and well-being:

- plan, monitor and evaluate health promotion strategies;
- plan, implement, monitor and evaluate prevention and screening programmes;
- protect population health by managing outbreaks, incidents and emergencies.

3 Developing quality and risk management within an evaluative culture:

- assess evidence of effectiveness of health interventions;
- improve quality through audit and evaluation;
- manage risk to public's health and well-being.

4 Collaborative working for health:

- develop and sustain cross-sectional working;
- communicate effectively with the public and others.

5 Developing health programmes and services and reducing inequalities:

- develop, implement and evaluate health programmes and services;
- facilitate the reduction of inequalities in health.

6 Policy and strategy development and implementation:

- shape and influence the development of health and social care policy;
- implement strategies to put policies into effect;
- assess impact of policies.

7 Working with and for communities:

- involve the public and communities as active partners;
- empower communities;
- advocate for communities.

8 Strategic leadership for health:

- develop, sustain and implement a vision and objectives for health;
- lead teams and individuals to improve health and reduce inequalities.

9 Research & Development:

- appraise, plan and manage research;
- develop and implement research findings in practice.

10 Ethically managing self, people and resources:

- manage the development and direction of work;
- develop capacity and capability to improve health;
- deliver effective services, the aim of which is to improve health.

(Taken and adapted from HDA Public Health Skills Audit (2001). Available at: www.hda-online.org.uk/downloads/pdfs/audit_tool_participants.pdf)

People can work in public health in a great variety of ways. Not everyone wants, or needs, to cover all the standards given above. However, the list of specialist standards provides a comprehensive and useful checklist from which to identify which public health skills you need for your particular role. It can also serve as a tool to help identify the range of complementary skills needed by a team of people with differing responsibilities for public health.

We suggest that you use the template below to reflect on your role and identify the skills that you require. You may consider areas where you already have skills, identify areas that you need to develop further and what action you will take to achieve that development. We hope that this book will prove helpful in achieving the progress that you wish to make.

Reflect on what your skills currently are, where there are gaps and any action arising.

Public health standards	
Surveillance & assessment	
Promoting & protecting	
Developing quality & risk management	
Collaborative working for health	
Developing programmes & services & reducing inequalities	
Policy & strategy development & implementation	
Working with & for communities	
Strategic leadership	
Research & Development	
Ethically managing self, people & resources	

1

Lessons from the history of public health and epidemiology for the twenty-first century

How do you define epidemiology and public health?

What have been other names public health has had in previous centuries?

Is disease caused by miasmas?

What information do you need to report the number of deaths per 10,000 population?

What were the driving forces to implement public health interventions in different centuries?

After working through this chapter you should be able to:

- illustrate through the use of historical data/examples how thinking regarding time–person–place evolved;
- define concepts underpinning the evolution of epidemiology and public health thinking, such as statistics, infectious disease epidemiology, disaster epidemiology, chronic disease epidemiology, molecular epidemiology, measures of risk and prediction of risk;
- place within a historical context public health successes as well as remaining and new challenges.

We start this introductory study guide to public health and epidemiology with a look back into history. We cover how the two concepts evolved over time and in different parts of the world. Before we provide you with current definitions we ask you to do an exercise on your own current understanding of what public health is.

Exercise 1.1

These are some of the terms that have been used for public health activity over time:

- State medicine
- Public health medicine
- Social medicine
- Hygiene
- Environmental health
- Community medicine
- Public medicine
- New public health
- Complete medical police

Give some thought to how this terminology may reflect scientific concepts about the causes of disease and health in their time. Also think about how the relationships between central government, local government (elected) and local authorities (appointed) and individuals may be reflected in these terms. Note your thoughts here.

Which in your view are the key terms that should appear in a contemporary definition of public health?

Defining what public health is

You may have considered that some of these definitions contain the term 'medicine' whereas others don't. This is a reflection of two contradictory directions that have pulled on public health as a discipline for centuries. One concept of public health is based on a broad focus on the underlying social and economic causes of health and disease and their variation in populations. The other has a narrower medical focus with treatment of ill health at its centre.

You have noticed the terms like 'state medicine' or 'complete medical police' which sound a bit awkward in this day and age. The organization of public health structures has always been closely related to the way communities and societies organize themselves, which role was allocated to the ruling class in looking after the well-being of citizens, which responsibilities were allocated to citizens themselves.

In the following we provide you with two modern definitions of what public health is about. The first is from the 1987 UK Acheson Report which looked into the future of the public health function: 'Public Health is the art and science of preventing disease, promoting health and prolonging life through organised efforts of society'. Beaglehole and Bonita's book *Public Health at the Crossroads*, published in 2004, defines public health as 'Collective action for sustained population-wide health improvement'.

Example of interagency working to protect public health

As an example of the roles of government bodies and local authorities in implementing public health measures, think of national standards for food with regards to contamination with unwanted micro-organisms, as well as chemical contaminants. Such standards are set by central government based on available evidence. Local authorities implement standards by regular inspection of premises that produce or sell food. They will, for example, check the temperature records of fridges and freezers as an indication that the cool chain has been maintained. Manufacturers of foods have to obtain a licence from a regulator and they have to put 'use by' dates on their produce. Consumers are advised to use the information on food labels to make choices about what they eat and when. This illustrates how today we are used to having a range of measures in place that make sure that the food we consume is fit for consumption.

Early history of public health practice

You may have already considered the role of the concept of disease being preventable as a central point of public health thinking. If diseases are known to be preventable, society may decide to give a role to certain public health professionals to make sure that people remain healthy for longer. This may either be prompted by concern for their health *per se* or by a desire to reduce poverty by keeping people healthy enough to work, or it could be prompted by a desire to keep civil order.

Chinese medicine, Ayurvedic medicine in India (400 BC), Hippocrates in Greece (460–377 BC) and Galen (AD 129–199) in Rome and their followers were aware of the influences of season, diet, the winds and lifestyle for individual people's health. Galen created the theory of 'miasma' or bad air causing disease. A miasma was seen as consisting of malodorous and poisonous particles created by decomposing organic matter. For hundreds of years the 'miasma' theory competed with the theory of contagion. This contagion theory had its origin in the success of the ancient practice of isolating ill people. The discovery of the microscope in 1683 was followed by the discovery of micro-organisms in the late nineteenth century. These dicoveries drastically changed the theory of disease causation and the 'contagion theory' dominated public health thinking between the late nineteenth century and the mid-twentieth century.

Theories of disease causation, disease being seen as preventable, together with a high level of organization of society, were required in designing systematic approaches to disease prevention. They were targeted at fighting the major disease outbreaks such as plagues and leprosy. Between 1347 and 1351 the plague or the 'Black Death' killed approximately one-third (23 million) of the total population of Europe's 80 million people within only a three-year period. While medical Islamic doctors had developed the science of hygiene to a very high level, they agreed with their Christian counterparts that plagues were God-given and should not be fought.

Public health after 1600

It was in the Italian city states such as Milan and Florence in the sixteenth century that the concepts of purification of enclosed space – quarantine, a 40-day hold on ships, and isolation of victims, washing surfaces with lime and vinegar – were developed for the protection of wealthy citizens. These cities also began providing 'lazarettes' to house plague victims and for the first time created semi-permanent public health posts to enforce plague regulations.

The concept of the dirtiness of air as being the root cause of disease outbreaks is reflected in two seventeenth-century documents from Britain: John Evelyn's

'*Fumifugium or the Inconvenience of the Air and Smoke of London Dissipated*' and John Graunt's '*The Nature and Political Observations made upon the Bills of Mortality*' (1662).

John Graunt (1620–74) wrote:

> When I consider, that in my country seventy are born for fifty eight buried, and that before 1600 the like happened in London, I considered whether a City, as it becomes more populous, doth not, for that very cause, become more unhealthfull, ... but chiefly, because I have heard, that 60 years ago few Sea-Coals were burnt in London, which now are universally used. For I have heard, that Newcastle is more unhealthfull than other places . . .

John Graunt links population growth to the increasing need for fuel. After the forests around London had been cut down, the resulting energy crisis was met by importing sea-coal from Newcatle in the north-east of England. Newcastle upon Tyne, the city of origin of sea-coal, is the city where this study guide is being written. This is one of the early accounts linking air pollution with the health of populations, in this case the residents of London and Newcastle.

Inventing and defining epidemiology

John Graunt also describes how parish clerks used weekly records of mortality to communicate with members of the public about the extent or absence of an epidemic.

This takes us to defining the second core discipline of this introductory study guide: Epidemiology. While epidemiology is still too often and too closely associated with the idea of fighting epidemics: epi (*upon*), demos (*the people*), and logos (*to study*), it actually incorporates much wider concepts.

Epidemiology is the study of the distribution and determinants of health-related states or events in human populations and the application of this study to the control of health problems. The core of epidemiology is the use of quantitative methods to study disease and risk factors in human populations. Epidemiology is a relatively young science only dating back to John Graunt and possibly a hundred years later to James Lind (1794).

James Lind was a British navy doctor. He is credited with designing the first ever clinical trial. He had the hypothesis that scurvy, a debilitating disease affecting sailors on long sea journeys, was caused by lack of fruit intake. He enrolled 12 sailors suffering from scurvy and split them into six different treatment groups. Those two sailors that were given two oranges and a lemon per day made an almost complete recovery. Other treatments included cider, sea water and vinegar. He published his study in 1753. Lind interpreted the results of his study to mean that oranges and lemons are a remedy for scurvy rather than a means of preventing it. It took many years until evidence had emerged that scurvy could be completely avoided if foods containing vitamin C were part of the provisions. From 1795 onwards limes were included in sailors' provisions in the UK. The legacy of this practice is still reflected in that present-day English sailors are called 'limeys'.

The registration of births and deaths is an essential prerequisite for monitoring disease rates in populations and for any comparisons between places. Sweden was the first country to introduce a national system of registration to monitor population growth and vital statistics in 1748, to promote fertility and personal hygiene. The next exercise (1.2) gives you some early health statistics from the UK including information about the place and the occupation of deceased people.

Exercise 1.2

Average age in years of deceased persons (Chadwick 1842)

Locality	Professional, Gentry	Tradesman	Labourers, Servants
Wiltshire (rural)	50	48	33
Derby (urban industrial)	49	38	21
Kensington (wealthy urban)	44	29	26
Leeds (urban industrial)	44	27	19
Liverpool (urban industrial sea port)	35	22	15

What observations can you make based on these early health statistics?

How did the occupations and the locality influence the age of the deceased?

How do these statistics compare with what you know about current health differentials in your own country and community?

Edwin Chadwick (1800–84) used the data given in Exercise 1.2 to advocate that saving the lives of breadwinners would be justified because it lowered the cost to society supporting widows and orphans. He advocated investment in comprehensive systems of water and sewage. Today we know that by focusing on bad sanitation as a universal cause of disease Chadwick's ideas deflected from other causes of disease such as malnutrition and long working hours. Poverty was seen as an effect of disease, not a cause.

There were also differences in approach between countries. In the UK, sanitation dominated public health thinking more than in other places. In France and America the concept of health as a right of their citizens in combination with the citizen's responsibility to maintain their own health was part of what is called the 'Enlightenment philosophy of democratic citizenship' which developed during the period 1760s to 1790s. As a consequence, the French Revolution incorporated a system of social assistance and free medical care. At the same time, Johann Peter Frank (1745–1821) in Germany advocated an authoritarian 'medical police' with a strong central role of the state in both provision and control of public services, which was not popular in Britain or America.

A contemporary of Edwin Chadwick, William Farr, who had studied in Paris, observed in 1866: 'No variation in the health of the states of Europe is the result of chance. It is the direct result of the physical and political conditions in which nations live.' Farr stressed the need for economic, environmental and social reform to improve health, a conclusion in direct contrast to Chadwick's.

A very successful early campaign of disease prevention was the inoculation against smallpox. This was brought to Europe by the wife of the British ambassador in Constantinople, now Istanbul in Turkey in 1718 (see Box 1.1 for a chronology of the eradication of smallpox).

Box 1.1 Public health success: the eradication of smallpox

1718 Lady Mary Watley Montague (1689–1762), wife of the British ambassador to Constantinople, reports on the common practice of inoculation in the Ottoman Empire.

1760s Inoculation commercially available.

1796 Dr E. Jenner's inoculation with cowpox (vaccinia virus) prevents smallpox.

1806 Thomas Jefferson (US President): 'Future nations will know by history only that the loathsome smallpox has existed'.

1853 Smallpox vaccination made compulsory for children under 5 in Britain.

1966 Global eradication of smallpox formulated as goal by World Health Organisation (WHO).

1977 Last national case of smallpox.

1980 WHO declares global eradication: 'the world and all its peoples have won freedom from smallpox, which was a most devastating disease sweeping many countries since earliest times leaving death, blindness and disfigurement in its wake'.

John Snow, a graduate from the very first batch of medical students from Newcastle upon Tyne, became famous for his investigations of the cholera epidemics in London in 1848–49 and 1853–54. Based on data in Exercise 1.3 he decided to remove the pump handle from a water pump which he saw as responsible for local residents getting infected with cholera (the Broad Street pump).

John Snow's action to remove the pathway of exposure happened at a time when microbes as agents of infectious diseases had not yet been identified. He therefore did not yet know that the cholera bacillus was required for people to get infected and that it was transmitted by sewage-contaminated drinking water. Given that the cholera epidemic had been raging for some time, which resulted in large population movements, the Census data from three years prior may no longer have been very accurate. Consequently the calculated rates may well have had gross errors.

The first era of epidemiology, based on engineering, hygiene and sanitation, came to an end in the late nineteenth century when bacteria were discovered. For more than 50 years thereafter both epidemiology and public health were dominated by what we call a bacteriological paradigm. Disease status was now defined by a laboratory-based diagnosis rather than a patient complaint. In parallel to this, public health became dominated by people in medical professions. New training schemes

---

Exercise 1.3

John Snow's cholera data from the London cholera epidemic in 1854

Water Company	Population in 1851 Census	Deaths from cholera in 14 weeks (end Oct 1854)	Deaths in 10,000 living
Southwark and Vauxhall (which includes the pump at Broad Street)	1263	4093	153
Lambeth	173,748	461	26
Rest of London	2,362,236	10,367	43

What observations can you make with regards to the death rates in the three areas of London?

Can you think of any weaknesses in the data that John Snow was using?

Source: *On the Mode of Communication of Cholera* (Reprinted in (1988) *The Challenges of Epidemiology*. Washington, DC: Pan American Health Organisation, pp. 42–5).

---

were developed in many countries to train such professionals. Alongside the medical label of disease status, diagnoses could carry social stigma and bring loss of employment even if somebody was a healthy carrier.

In Exercise 1.4 you will be introduced to the concept of diseases being caused by a range of factors, which may or may not include an infectious agent. You already know that the disease tuberculosis is caused by the tubercle bacillus. Now have a look at Exercise 1.4 and see whether that is strictly speaking true.

You may have considered a range of factors that impact on the likelihood of people:

1 being infected with mycobacterium tuberculosis;
2 becoming ill with tuberculosis; and
3 dying from tuberculosis after having been infected and shown signs of disease.

Hygiene and overcrowded housing are two factors which influence the likelihood of becoming infected. Overcrowding, in turn, is influenced by family size and reproductive behaviour. Two factors that influence how serious tuberculosis is for an infected individual are nutritional status and personal hygiene. Personal hygiene depends on whether you know how about personal hygiene and then whether you have the means to carry it out. How well nourished you are depends on your knowledge about healthy food and how well off you are. Access to medical care is of course another important factor in determining whether you are likely to get better after contracting the disease. The introduction of the antibiotic streptomycine and the

Exercise 1.4

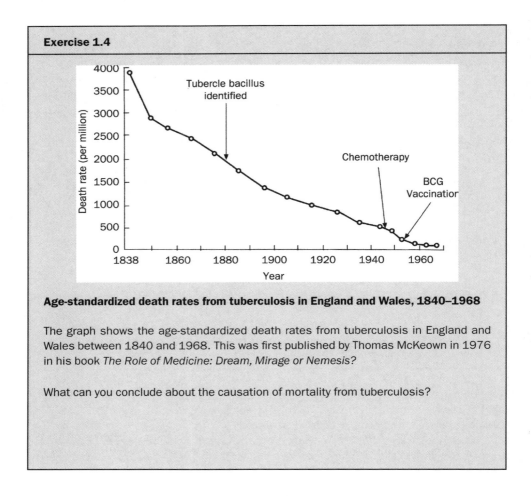

Age-standardized death rates from tuberculosis in England and Wales, 1840–1968

The graph shows the age-standardized death rates from tuberculosis in England and Wales between 1840 and 1968. This was first published by Thomas McKeown in 1976 in his book *The Role of Medicine: Dream, Mirage or Nemesis?*

What can you conclude about the causation of mortality from tuberculosis?

tuberculosis (BCG) vaccine do not seem to have made a great impact on the overall tuberculosis mortality.

Non-communicable disease: epidemiology and public health in the twentieth century

While early epidemiology was dominated by infectious diseases, the early twentieth century saw some consideration of non-infectious causes of disease. The American Joseph Goldberger concluded in 1914 and then in 1930 that pellagra was not an infectious disease but was due to diet (later determined as lack of vitamin B). In the past 50 years many investigations linking non-communicable diseases with health outcomes have centred around personal behaviours, often couched as behaviour choices. Such behaviours in turn have been the focus of much public health practice (smoking, alcohol intake, obesity, levels of physical activity). Epidemiological studies have made great contributions towards unravelling the complex interplay of a range of risk factors. However, they have often failed to consider broader environmental and social determinants of health behaviour. Many prevention programmes have taken the form of blaming and stigmatizing individuals for their unhealthy habits without considering wider social factors that underpin lifestyle choices.

The final exercise (1.5) introduces you to one of the key studies which identified smoking as a key risk factor for lung cancer. The study investigated the link between

---

Exercise 1.5

In England and Wales the phenomenal increase in the number of deaths attributed to cancer of the lung provides one of the most striking changes in the pattern of mortality recorded by the Registrar-General. For example, in the quarter of a century between 1922 and 1947 the annual number of deaths recorded increased from 612 to 9287, or roughly fifteen-fold. This remarkable increase is, of course, out of all proportion to the increase of population – both in total and, particularly, in its older age groups. Stocks, using standardized death rates to allow for these population changes, show the follow-ing trend: rate per 100 000 in 1901–1920, males 1.1, females 0.7; rate per 100 000 in 1936–1939, males 10.6, females 2.5. The rise seems to have been particularly rapid since the end of the First World War: between 1921–1930 and 1940–1944 the death rate of men at ages 45 and over increased six-fold and of women of the same ages approximately threefold. This increase is still continuing. It has occurred too, in Switzerland, Denmark, the USA, Canada and Australia and has been reported from Turkey and Japan.

Two main causes have from time to time been put forward: (1) a general atmos-pheric pollution from the exhaust fumes of cars, from the surface dust of tarred roads and from gasworks, industrial plants and coal fires; and (2) the smoking of tobacco

Number of cases	Number of cigarettes smoked daily (maximum)			
	1 cig. %	5 cig. %	15 cig. %	25+ cig. %
Males				
Lung cancer patients (647)	3.7	32.1	30.3	33.9
Control patients (622)	6.1	38.9	32.3	22.7
Females				
Lung cancer patients (41)	14.6	36.6	29.3	19.5
Control patients (28)	42.9	32.1	21.4	3.6

What observations can you make regarding the link between smoking and lung cancer from the data in the table above?

What alternative explanations would you have considered for the findings?

Source: Doll, R. and Bradford Hill, A. (1950) Smoking and carcinoma of the lung: preliminary report, *British Medical Journal*, 30 September, pp. 739–48.

smoking and lung cancer in 20 London hospitals between April 1948 and October 1949. It was published in 1950.

Here are extracts from the original paper to let you know how the authors interpreted their findings:

> From the table it will be seen that apart from the general excess of smokers found in lung-carcinoma patients, there is in this group a significantly higher proportion of heavier smokers and a correspondingly lower proportion of lighter smokers than in the comparative group of other patients. For instance, in the lung-carcinoma group 33.9 per cent of the male patients fall in the group of highest consumption (25 cigarettes a day or more), while in the control group of other male patients only 22.7 per cent are found there. The same trend is observable for women.

Interpretation of Results

Though from the table in Exercise 1.5 there seems to be no doubt that there is a direct association between smoking and carcinoma of the lung, it is necessary to consider alternative explanations of the results. Could they be due to an unrepresentative sample of patients with carcinoma of the lung or to a choice of a control series which was not truly comparable? Could they have been produced by an exaggeration of their smoking habits by patients who thought they had an illness which could be attributed to smoking? Could they be produced by bias on the part of the interviewers in taking and interpreting the histories?

To summarize, it is not reasonable, in our view, to attribute the results to any special selection of cases or to bias in recording. In other words, it must be concluded that there is a real association between carcinoma of the lung and smoking. Many subsequent studies have confirmed this.

Molecular and genetic epidemiology and biological monitoring

Over the past 20 years or so a range of molecular techniques have been added to the portfolio that epidemiologists use to link exposure with disease information.

Measuring a potentially harmfully substance in blood, urine, or teeth allows one to consider jointly all routes of exposure, be it inhalation, uptake via food and water (oral) or via the skin (dermal). Measuring the early response within a critical target organ is conceptually a very attractive way of improving the quality of exposure assessment. However, in practice, the applications of biomarkers of exposure have been much more limited for a number of reasons. These include their often short biological half-life which means that only exposure in the recent past can be investigated. Often it is not yet well understood what the markers are actually measuring.

The role of individual susceptibility to cancer-causing agents and the development of molecular techniques to identify individual strains of bacteria through by their genome sequence promised a big surge in the proportion of explained disease variation some years back.

However, even for such an intensely studied disease as breast cancer the currently six identified genes explain only approximately 20 per cent of the aggregation of breast cancer in families.

In the developed world it is likely that molecular and genetic epidemiology and biological monitoring research will continue for quite a while. In terms of methods for improving global public health, it is much more likely, that broad public health evidence-based measures such as the millennium development goals on child mortality, maternal health, environment sustainability, poverty and gender equality will impact much more on the global burden of disease.

In parallel to the changing paradigms and theories that have underpinned public health practice and epidemiology, there have also been changes in the nature of the evidence that impacts on public health practice. These aspects will be covered in some more detail in the final chapter of the book (Chapter 11).

Summary

Working through the chapter should have helped you to answer the questions posed at the beginning. You can use the following headings to summarize the most important aspects of the chapter for you:

1   Give a definition of epidemiology and public health.

2   Write down other names public health has had over time and the reasons why those names were given.

3   Compare and contrast the miasma and contagion concepts of disease causation.

4   Write notes on two of the case studies covered, reflecting on what the driving forces were for the implementation of public health interventions.

Now reflect again on what your skills and knowledge currently are, where there are gaps and any actions arising.

Public health standards	
Surveillance & assessment	
Promoting & protecting	
Developing quality & risk management	
Collaborative working for health	
Developing programmes & services & reducing inequalities	
Policy & strategy development & implementation	
Working with & for communities	
Strategic leadership	
Research & Development	
Ethically managing self, people & resources	

2

Sources and critical use of health information

What types of information are needed to inform public health practice?

How should the quality of routinely available health information be judged?

In the absence of routinely available health information what approaches may be used?

What cautions need to be exercised in comparing differences in health information over time or between places?

After working through this chapter, you should be able to:

- provide an overview of the different types of information that are relevant to public health practice;
- give an account of the types of information that tend to be routinely available on population characteristics, fertility, morbidity and mortality;
- provide a set of guidelines on the critical use of routinely available health information;
- suggest approaches to the collection of health information that may be used in situations where they are not routinely available;
- discuss the concept of the 'health care iceberg';
- critically compare health information collected in different places or at different points in time.

What types of health information do we need and what is routinely available?

The term 'information' is used to refer to a collection of facts, or items of data, that are meaningful. Public health is concerned with the protection and the improvement of the health of populations and communities. A huge variety of information is required to guide public health practice, which can be seen as having three broad elements (see Figure 2.1):

- understanding public health problems;
- setting priorities and developing interventions to address those problems; and
- the implementation of interventions to tackle the public health problems.

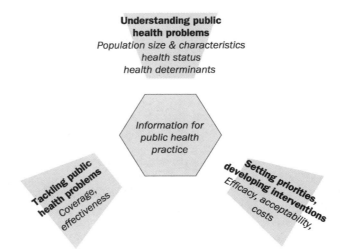

Figure 2.1 Examples of the types of information required for public health practice

Clearly many types of information are required for each of these elements. These will be highlighted throughout the book, with the last chapter (Chapter 11) aiming to provide an overview of how public health moves from understanding public health problems through to implementing and monitoring the impact of interventions to tackle those problems.

This chapter is concerned with some of the core information that is required to understand and monitor the public health, which is essential, although not enough, for public health practice. Consider the types of information that might be needed to describe the health status and determinants of health of a community by working through Exercise 2.1.

Factors you may have considered under 'determinants' include:

- *Influences to do with the individual* – for example, behavioural factors such as smoking, diet and exercise; knowledge and attitudes to health issues; wealth, employment and educational background; personality and response to stressful situations.
- *Influences to do with the local social, economic and physical environment* – for example, levels of crime and vandalism; the quality of housing; access to health care; access to good food; access to leisure facilities; levels of traffic and road

---

Exercise 2.1

Consider the local area in which you live: depending on your circumstances this might mean a street of houses, a hall of residence, a block of flats or an area of a village or town. You have been asked to describe the health and the determinants of health for residents in your area. List the information you would seek to obtain.

1　To describe the health of the residents

2　To describe the determinants (influences on) the health of the residents (you could break this down into influences to do with the individual; with the local social, economic and physical environment; and with the wider social, economic and physical environment).

In describing the health status of residents in your area you may have started by wanting to know their number by age and sex, as both of these can have major implications for health. You may have mentioned deaths and causes of death and episodes of illness. You may also have mentioned more positive aspects of health, perhaps trying to define general well-being and quality of life.

---

traffic accidents; employment and educational opportunities in the area; levels of air pollution.

- *Influences to do with the wider social, economic, and physical environment* – for example, advertising and pricing policy on tobacco and alcohol; road safety legislation; legislation on contraception and abortion; national economic and employment policy; the distribution of wealth; the effects of greenhouse gases and global warming.

We have covered some of the information we might like to collect to describe the health status of a community and the factors influencing that community's health. How much of this information is routinely available? 'Routinely available' refers to information that is collected, collated (put together and analysed), and is disseminated on a regular basis. The answer, of course, depends partly on where you are. In the sections that follow, the major types of routinely available information that are available in most rich countries, such as those of Western Europe and North America, are described. These major types include information on the following:

- The size, age and sex structure, ethnicity and socio-economic characteristics of the population.
- Rates of births and deaths, and causes of death.
- Episodes of illness and disease.
- In addition, a variety of other information relevant to health is often routinely available, from rates of specific health care interventions, such as immunization and screening, to areas such as routine monitoring of air quality.

Before considering these sources of information we will consider issues to do with using such information critically.

Using information critically

There is a lot of information around which is relevant to health. The information which is available, however, is a very mixed bag, of varying quality and usefulness. Any source of information must be used critically. Here are four areas you should consider:

- *Validity or appropriateness* – Is the information a true expression of what you are interested in? For example, if you were interested in the amount of lung cancer in the community, then looking at the number of deaths from lung cancer should give a reasonable idea because most people with lung cancer die from it within a fairly short space of time. What if you were interested in the amount of diabetes in the community? Deaths from diabetes would give a very poor impression of this. Diabetes is a chronic condition with very long average duration. Although the majority of people with diabetes die from one of its complications, which include coronary heart disease and stroke, diabetes is frequently not recorded as a cause of death.

- *Accuracy* – How carefully and precisely was the information collected and recorded; are there likely to be errors, and if so, what are the nature of those errors? Inaccuracies can arise at several points. For example, if the information is based on hospital records, how accurate was the original information in the hospital records, and how accurately was that information coded, transcribed and turned into routine statistics?

- *Completeness* – Does the information cover all the individuals or all the events that you are interested in? Completeness refers to whether all the information is recorded on each person as well as whether everyone who should be (or every event) is included.

- *Timeliness* – Was the information collected recently enough to be useful? How up to date the information needs to be depends on what you want to use it for. Information that is one or two years old on the size and characteristics of a population is likely to be perfectly acceptable (barring major social upheaval over that time) to describe such things as the age, sex, ethnic mix, types of housing, and so on; information of this age to monitor levels of food poisoning would be useless – the picture could easily have changed over this time, but just as importantly the time scale would be far too long to allow effective preventive action to be taken.

Consider the issues of validity, accuracy, completeness, timeliness for an information source with which you are familiar in Exercise 2.2 (facing).

Information on population size and characteristics

A census is a count, an enumeration, of the population. One of the most famous censuses is that reported in the *New Testament* following a 'decree from Caesar

---

Exercise 2.2

As a health care worker or student you are likely to have been a collector of health information, such as through contributions to patient or client records. Choose one of the areas to which you have contributed. Write below what you know about the accuracy, completeness and timeliness of the information.

Could this information source be used to help build up a picture of the health of the local community? Give your reasons, including reservations you may have about the use of the information in this way.

Augustus that all the world should be enrolled' and that is why Mary and Joseph travelled to Bethlehem.

Most rich and many low and middle income countries undertake regular censuses of their populations. The usual aim of census enumeration is to record the identity of every person in every place of residence, including their age or date of birth, sex, marital status and occupation. Other personal details may also be recorded such as place of birth, race or ethnicity, educational history, literacy and general health status. Details on living conditions, such as the number of rooms in the house and the type of toilet are also frequently collected. In most countries the census is the main source of information on the size, age and sex structure and basic socio-economic characteristics of the population.

As an example we will describe the census in the United Kingdom. Regular ten yearly censuses have been carried out since 1801, with one omission which was in 1941 (in the midst of the Second World War). Details of the census procedures, and its results, can be found through the Office of National Statistics (web address at the end of this chapter). During the last census, in 2001, information was collected about households, as well as about individuals. Data were collected on age, sex, marital status, ethnicity, occupation and employment, education, car ownership, housing tenure and the presence of long-standing illness.

For the administration of the census the whole country is divided into enumeration districts (in other countries similar administrative units are often called 'census tracts'). On average each enumeration district contains about 200 households. An enumerator is responsible for ensuring that a form is delivered to every household prior to the night of the census and is collected from that household as soon after the census as possible. The head of the household is required by law to provide details on the census form for every person who is a member of the household, present or absent, on the night of the census.

Now that you know a little about the census in the UK and how it is conducted, think through some of the issues of accuracy, completeness and timeliness by working through Exercise 2.3.

The accuracy of the information is dependent on the people completing the form i.e. the heads of household. The head of household may not be familiar with all the

---

Exercise 2.3

Under the following headings suggest potential shortcomings of census information:

• Accuracy

• Completeness

• Timeliness

---

details required on other individuals in the household. He/she may use vague terms for such items as occupation, making it difficult to put the individuals into a definite occupational category when the ONS come to code and analyse the data. The census aims to count every person living in the United Kingdom on the night of the census. It obtains information about those not present at their residence from the head of the household. However, some people will not be counted in a census, others will be counted twice. In terms of health needs, a major concern is those people without a permanent address, for example, those living in temporary accommodation, and those sleeping rough. We know that these people have specific health needs, but the census will only count a small proportion of them. Despite the legal requirement some people, particularly in inner city areas, may refuse to complete the census form. Finally, in terms of timeliness, it is a major drawback of the census that it occurs only once every ten years. Estimates of the population between censuses are based on births, deaths and migrations. The first two are accurately known, but internal migration (i.e., within the UK) is hard to track in many countries and so population estimates for small areas, particularly where migration is high, may become quite inaccurate over this time. Similarly, the social and economic fabric of an area can change markedly in ten years.

Information on fertility and mortality

Registration of vital events

There are several possible sources of information on fertility and mortality, such as hospital and maternity records and data collected as part of a census. The main source, however, in all rich countries, and many others, is from a system of registration of births and deaths. Such registration involves the creation of a permanent record for a birth or death. These records have a variety of uses within society. They include legal and civic uses, such as for establishing citizenship, rights to welfare services, and inheritance, through to areas that we are interested in here, such as monitoring trends in birth rates and death rates. The situation in the UK is described as an example although the system is very similar in all rich countries.

It has been a legal requirement since the nineteenth century that all births and deaths in the UK are registered. Throughout the country there is a network of Registry Offices where information on all births and deaths occurring in that area are collected. Each Registry Office is headed by a local registrar, a person who is appointed by the local government.

Registration of births and information on fertility

All births should be registered within 42 days by a parent or other informant. The information collected for the registration includes date and place of birth, the baby's first and last name, its sex and the name, address and place of birth of the parents, or just the mother if the father's details are not available. The birth registration data are made available to the Office of National Statistics which uses them, in conjunction with its demographic data from the census, to produce a series of statistics on fertility, some of which are detailed in Table 2.1.

Table 2.1 Definitions of some commonly used and readily available vital statistics

Statistic	Definition
Births and fertility	
Crude birth rate	Number of live births to residents of an area in one year per 1000 population of that area (usually based on the population present at the mid-year).
General fertility rate	Number of live births to residents of an area in one year per 1000 female population aged 15–44 years in that area.
Total period fertility rate	Average number of children per woman based on current fertility rates.
Mortality	
Perinatal mortality rate	Number of still births and deaths within the first week of life per 1000 total births (live and still) for a given year.
Infant mortality rate	Number of deaths in children under 1 year per 1000 live births for a given year.
Crude death rate	Number of deaths to residents of an area in one year per 1000 population of that area.
Age-specific death rate	Number of deaths to residents of an area in one age group in one year per 1000 population in that age group.
Cause-specific death rate	Number of deaths to residents of an area from a specific cause in one year per 1000 population.

Registration of deaths and information on mortality

When a death occurs, the registered medical practitioner who attended the deceased during their final illness is required by law to issue a medical certificate on the cause of death. The format for the certificate used was laid down in 1927, and the same basic format is recommended for international use. The certificate has two main sections (see Box 2.1). In section 1 of the certificate the doctor enters the conditions which led directly to death, with the disease or condition that started the sequence of events entered on the lowest line. Any other significant conditions that may have contributed to death are put in section 2.

The medical practitioner gives the death certificate to a 'qualified informant'.

Box 2.1 Internationally agreed format for indicating cause of death on death certificates

1 (a) Disease or condition directly leading to death_____

   (b) Other disease or condition, if any, leading to 1(a)_____

   (c) Other disease or condition, if any, leading to 1(b)_____

2 Other significant conditions contributing to the death but not related to the disease or condition causing it_____

This is usually a close relative of the deceased but could also be somebody like the person in charge of a rest home if that's where the deceased last resided. It is the responsibility of the qualified informant to take the death certificate to the local registrar's office to notify the death, and this should normally be done within five days of death. When they hand in the doctor's death certificate they will also be asked to provide the following information on the deceased: date and place of death; sex; usual address; full name, and maiden name if a married woman; date and place of birth; and occupation. If the registrar is satisfied (in some cases, such as a death in suspicious circumstances, the case may need to go to a coroner for cause of death to be determined), then all these details are forward to the ONS. At the ONS cause of death is coded. Most of the coding is done automatically by computer. The coding follows an internationally agreed system, called the International Classification of Diseases (or ICD for short), the latest version of which is the 10th revision (ICD–10).

Statistics on cause of death are almost always based on the underlying cause, as this tends to be the most useful for public health purposes. The World Health Organization defines the underlying cause of death as follows:

1   The disease or injury which initiated the train of events directly leading to death.

2   The circumstances of the accident or violence which produced the fatal injury.

As long as the death certificate has been properly completed, the 'underlying cause' is that given in the lowest line of section 1. The whole process, from death to becoming a mortality statistic, is summarized in Figure 2.2.

Statistics on death rates and causes of death are one of the main sources used to describe the state of health of a population or community. Table 2.1 provides definitions of some of the readily available and commonly used mortality statistics. However, clearly for the purpose of describing the health of a population or community, mortality statistics have some major shortcomings. Give some thought to these by working through Exercise 2.4.

There are two major areas for inaccuracies in mortality data. One is in ascribing cause of death. It can often be very difficult to ascribe a single cause of death, never mind trying to break it down into a sequence of events from underlying cause leading to the immediate cause. This especially true in elderly people where the presence of several disease processes at once is quite possible. It is generally the case that with

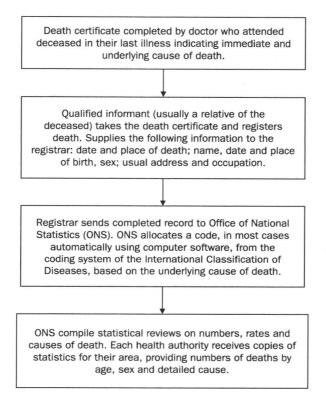

Death certificate completed by doctor who attended deceased in their last illness indicating immediate and underlying cause of death.

Qualified informant (usually a relative of the deceased) takes the death certificate and registers death. Supplies the following information to the registrar: date and place of death; name, date and place of birth, sex; usual address and occupation.

Registrar sends completed record to Office of National Statistics (ONS). ONS allocates a code, in most cases automatically using computer software, from the coding system of the International Classification of Diseases, based on the underlying cause of death.

ONS compile statistical reviews on numbers, rates and causes of death. Each health authority receives copies of statistics for their area, providing numbers of deaths by age, sex and detailed cause.

Figure 2.2 A summary of how mortality statistics are collected, collated and disseminated in England and Wales

---

Exercise 2.4

Under the following headings suggest potential shortcomings of cause of death information:

- Accuracy

- Completeness

- Timeliness

Are there any circumstances you can think of in which cause of death figures will provide a valid reflection of the health of a community or population?

increasing age of the deceased, the accuracy of the recorded cause of death decreases. The other major area for inaccuracies is in the information received by the registrar from the qualified informant. The accuracy of the information they give will depend on how well they knew the deceased, and may also be affected by their emotional state at the time. It is known, for example, that there can be an almost natural tendency to emphasize at such a time the importance of the deceased which could result in his/her occupation being embellished.

One of the advantages of death statistics, at least in most rich countries, compared to other forms of health statistics is that they are virtually 100 per cent complete. In many lower income countries deaths are very incompletely registered, and in such situations special studies need to be undertaken to find accurate estimates of death rates and cause of death. In terms of timeliness, it depends on their use. Mortality statistics in the UK for example appear within one year (or less) of being collected. This is quite adequate for most uses. However, obviously if you were using mortality statistics to identify epidemics of infectious diseases to which you wanted to make a rapid response, such as an outbreak of cholera, a year would be most untimely.

Finally, what were your views in Exercise 2.4 on the use of cause of death figures as a reflection of the health of a community? You may have answered that mortality can never adequately indicate health because health is much more than the absence of disease. This is a fair viewpoint. Yet, where death rates are very high, as they are in all ages in Sub-Saharan Africa, this is at least a pretty good indication that health is also very poor. Nonetheless, in both rich and poor country settings there are some major causes of ill health that make little direct contribution to mortality. These include mental health problems and diseases of the bones and joints. Attempts have been made, described later in this chapter, to produce a combined measure of mortality and morbidity so that using a single figure the overall health (or more correctly, ill health) status of two populations might be compared.

Information on the causes of morbidity and the health care iceberg

Routinely available information on morbidity comes mainly from data on the activity of health services. In theory, such information ought to provide a much better indication of the causes of ill health in a community than information on mortality. Unfortunately this promise is rarely realized. The types of morbidity data that are available vary greatly between different countries, tend to change as health care structures change and change in response to changing approaches to collecting, analysing and disseminating the information.

The aim here therefore is not to describe any of the systems for collecting morbidity in detail but to highlight issues in the use and interpretation of such information. One issue which is common to any data source based on health care activity is what has been called the health care iceberg. This is illustrated in Figure 2.3. People admitted to hospital represent only the tip of the iceberg of all people who are ill in the community. Even using the best information from primary health care will miss a significant proportion of people who are ill, who may not seek help or may seek the advice of friends, relatives, pharmacists or alternative therapists rather than members

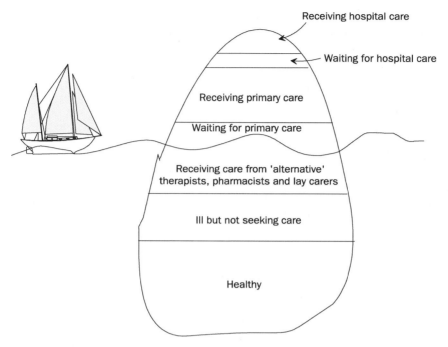

Figure 2.3 Illustration of the health care 'iceberg'
Source: Based on an illustration in Donaldson and Donaldson (1983) *Essential Community Medicine*. Cambridge, MA: MTP Press.

of the primary health care team. It will also of course miss people who have a disease but who do not feel ill, such as can be case in early cancer, heart disease, diabetes and many other diseases.

As examples of routinely available morbidity data, we will briefly consider three sources available within the UK, but typical of the situation in many other rich countries as well.

Infectious disease notification

Doctors are required by law to inform a local medical officer for infectious disease control if they suspect that a patient is suffering from one of around 30 infectious diseases. These diseases include measles, meningitis, tuberculosis, whooping cough, cholera and food poisoning. The aim of this system is to allow the local medical officer to take appropriate action to prevent further cases of the disease. Thus accuracy of diagnosis is considered less important than speed, as the diagnosis can always be checked once the notification is made. Unfortunately, although infectious disease notification is a legal requirement, underreporting is very common. Even with diseases which almost always require hospitalization, such as meningococcal meningitis, up to 50 per cent of cases may not be reported. Thus notifications tend to be incomplete and many will be inaccurate. Despite this, they seem to be adequate for following major trends and identifying outbreaks, the assumption being that if levels of underreporting and accuracy remain the same, then changes in the number of notifications represent a real change in the amount of disease. In England and Wales national figures on infectious disease notifications are collated, analysed and published by the Communicable Disease Surveillance Centre, CDSC. This centre monitors trends nationally, and is responsible for producing routine data on infectious disease notifications.

Cancer registration

Disease registers, which ideally contain the details of every person with a particular disease living in a geographically defined area, offer many potential rewards by providing high quality information for research, planning and patient management. Examples of diseases for which registers exist in some areas include diabetes, coronary heart disease and cancers. Cancer registries exist in many countries. A national cancer registration scheme was set up in the UK in 1962, and in each region there is a cancer registry covering a population usually of several million people. Cancer registration is not a legal requirement and the registry depends upon the cooperation of local doctors to inform them of patients with cancer. The registry also receives copies of death certificates of residents in their area on which cancer was mentioned as a cause of death. Registers require a huge amount of work, first, to try and identify every individual with the disease in the area, and, second, to keep the details of those on the register up to date. Studies of cancer registries in the UK suggest underreporting can be large, but that for those cases on the register the accuracy of the information is high.

Hospital activity data

In the UK these data are available from several different sources. Hospital Episode Statistics (as they are called in England) provide one of the main sources. An episode of treatment refers to a period of care received under one particular hospital consultant. If an individual is transferred to the care of another consultant, this counts as a new episode. If an individual was discharged and readmitted ten times in one year, this would be recorded as ten episodes and would be indistinguishable on the statistics from ten individuals each admitted once. Thus episodes of care, not individuals, are the basic unit being counted. Since 1997 it has become possible, in theory at least, to track individuals in the Hospital Episode Statistics by using the NHS number which is unique for each individual. However, at the time of writing this number is often not available in the data that have been entered. From each hospital, a minimum data set for each episode is sent to the Department of Health for collation into national statistics on hospital activity. Data collected in the hospital episode information system include the speciality of the consultant under whose care the episode took place, the clinical diagnosis, the admission and discharge date, the referring general practitioner and the age, sex and usual address of the patient. Hospital episode statistics are a potentially very useful source of information about illnesses treated in hospital. Their actual usefulness, however, in providing a basis for the assessment of health service needs has been disputed, mainly because of the quality of the diagnostic information and its completeness. In addition, factors other than rates of illness may determine differences between hospitals or areas. Such factors include differences in the number of beds available, admission policies, average distance to the hospital and referral practices. Finally, activity in private hospitals is not included, which in some areas is a substantial part of the health care used by residents.

This brief overview of morbidity data illustrates some of the major problems in their collection and use. Completeness and accuracy are recurring themes, and a striking drawback of hospital activity data is that episodes are counted rather than individuals (although this problem could be solved by using unique personal identifiers to track individuals). You have probably also picked up from discussion of the three examples above that the systems are quite separate. Being able to link these systems together routinely (this can be done after a huge effort in 'one-off' studies) would provide some major advantages. This is called *record linkage*. It requires that each individual has a unique and reliable personal identifier, such as an ID number. This identifier would have to be used on every information system, whether for disease notification, disease registration, hospital admissions, or at death registration. All of these information systems would then need to be brought together (which in practical terms means on the same computer system in a common format). With such a system it would be possible do such things as count the number of sick individuals in a population based on the information available and to follow individuals through courses of hospital treatment. In some countries individuals are given a unique identifying number at birth which is then used on all health records. This greatly facilitates record linkage, and even without routinely bringing all the data together onto one system, ad hoc record linkage studies are much easier. Of course, being able to link individual's records together in this way also raises the huge ethical and political issues, to do with patient confidentiality and potential abuses of the information.

Other routinely available information relevant to health

Above we have considered routinely available information on population size and characteristics, fertility, mortality and aspects of morbidity. In addition to these areas there may be many others types of routinely available information that are relevant to health. Examples of the types of other routinely available information in the UK are given in Table 2.2.

Approaches to obtaining information in situations where the data are not routinely available

In many parts of the world routinely available data of the type described above on population size and characteristics, births and deaths, and episodes of illness and disease, are not available. Or if they are available, they often suffer from serious problems of incompleteness or inaccuracy that render them not very useful. Various approaches have been used to provide types of data in such situations. They include demographic surveillance, epidemiological surveys, and rapid assessment methods.

Table 2.2 Examples of routinely available information relevant to health in the United Kingdom

---

Demographic information

Census information (includes numbers by age, sex and ethnicity, type of employment, educational level, house tenure, overcrowding . . .) for the area.

Births – details of all births registered in area, including birth weight and occupation of mother, etc.

Deaths – details of all deaths registered in the area, such as age, cause of death, place of death, occupation of deceased.

Population estimates and projections – estimates of population size between censuses, projected population size in future.

Vital statistics

Rates of deaths, including perinatal and infant mortality, birth rates and fertility rates.

Morbidity

Notifiable diseases – infectious disease notifications by age, sex, address, date organism.

Cancer registrations – diagnosis, age, sex, occupation, area of residence, details of treatment.

Hospital activity – by age, sex, method of admission, diagnosis, operative procedures, etc.

Socio-economic data

Unemployment benefit – numbers claiming by area.

Free school meals – numbers claiming by area.

Housing benefit – numbers claiming by area.

Income support – numbers claiming by area.

Environmental data

Road accidents – casualties and type of accident by area (police division), only includes accidents to which police are called.

Crime statistics – numbers and type of reported crime by area.

Air pollution – results from different monitoring sites around the city.

Drinking water – levels of lead and coliform bacteria by water supply zones.

Noise – number of complaints.

Pests – number of complaints for cockroaches, rats, etc.

Source: Lord, J. (1992) *A Guide to Data Sources in Manchester*. Manchester: Manchester Public Health and Human Resource Centre.

Some of the main characteristics and uses of these approaches are summarized in Table 2.3 (page 32).

Box 2.2 illustrates by way of example a national demographic surveillance system that has been established in Tanzania. This system aims to provide estimates of the burden of disease in Tanzania, including cause-specific mortality, and the major determinants of that disease burden, particularly its relationship to poverty. The information generated by the system is used in national policy-making, planning, and evaluation. The system also provides an invaluable infrastructure for undertaking other types of studies, such as on levels of morbidity from particular health problems.

Epidemiological survey methods are described in Chapter 5. Further reading for rapid evaluation methods can be found at the end of this chapter. Data from the demographic surveillance system in Tanzania are referred to again in subsequent chapters.

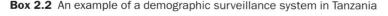

Box 2.2 An example of a demographic surveillance system in Tanzania

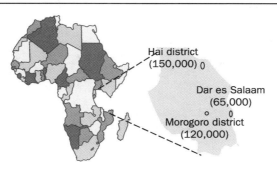

Hai district
(150,000) o

Dar es Salaam
(65,000)
o   0
Morogoro district
(120,000)

The surveillance sites:

Hai and Morogoro are rural areas, and Dar es Salaam is the major city in Tanzania. Numbers in brackets show the total, all ages, population (rounded to nearest 5000) under surveillance in 2001. These sites have been under surveillance since 1992. More recently a further 3 sites have been added to create a nationally representative surveillance system.

The methods:

- Annual censuses are carried out in the rural areas, and twice yearly in the urban area (because of higher migration). Networks of village and neighbourhood reporters record deaths on a continuous basis.
- Trained health care workers follow up each death and administer a 'verbal autopsy' interview with the next of kin and carers of the deceased person. Where they exist, medical records for the deceased are also obtained.
- Cause of death is assigned by a panel of three physicians, who do this independently of each other. Agreement between two is necessary to assign the cause of death.
- Information on births and migration is obtained from the censuses.

Note: For more information, see: www.ncl.ac.uk/ammp

Comparing routinely collected information over time and between areas

The main aim of this chapter has been to try and show the importance of a critical (some might even say sceptical) approach to using routinely available health information. Let's finish off with a very common scenario – making comparisons between areas, or over time. A good idea in using any information source is to try and think through the process involved from the data being collected to it being presented in its current form. Try and identify each step in the process and ask yourself what errors could arise at each step. Try doing this now when answering the questions in Exercise 2.5.

Table 2.3 Examples of ad hoc approaches to obtaining information on population size and characteristics, births and deaths, and episodes of disease and illness

Approach	Characteristics	Examples of uses
Demographic surveillance	Regular censuses of community or sub-section of a population. Systems for identifying births and deaths. May include system for ascribing cause of death.	Population size, age and sex structure; migration in and out of the population; measures of fertility and mortality; and provides an infrastructure for undertaking other ad hoc studies.
Epidemiological surveys	Representative sample of larger population selected. Survey participants interviewed and/or examined.	Assesses the prevalence of a disease; may be used to estimate fertility and mortality.
Rapid evaluation methods	Variety of methods may be used, such as: • participant observation; • focus group discussions; • key informant interviews; • patients interviews; and • health staff interviews.	Can provide a qualitative assessment of the major health problems, their causes and solutions. Commonly used to assess quality of health care delivery.

Exercise 2.5

In the following hypothetical comparisons assume that in reality there is no difference in the frequency of the disease. Try and think of some possible explanations for the apparent differences.

1   In the City of Manchester there has been a 50% increase in food poisoning notifications over 6 months.

2   Based on cancer registration data one area of the UK has a higher rate of bowel cancer than another area.

3   In two neighbouring health districts death rates from diabetes are substantially higher in one compared to the other.

For each of the hypothetical comparisons in Exercise 2.5 there are several possible explanations. Here are some suggestions.

1   Assuming levels of food poisoning in the city have stayed the same, then the most likely explanation is an increase in ascertainment. Perhaps the local medical officer recently ran a campaign to encourage all doctors to notify cases of food poisoning.

2   The most likely explanation is that in the area with the lower rate fewer of the cases are being notified to the cancer registry.

3   Remember that cause of death is based on the underlying cause given on the death certificate. A possible explanation is that in the district with the higher rate there is a team with a special interest in diabetes. If someone with diabetes dies of an immediate cause only possibly related to diabetes, they tend nevertheless to record it as the underlying cause of death, whereas in the other district diabetes would not be given as the underlying cause in this situation.

Summary

Write your own summary of this chapter by answering the following questions:

1   Summarize the range of routinely available information which may be useful in describing the health and determinants of health of a community or population.

2   Suggest four criteria with which to critically assess any information source.

3   Briefly describe the process by which deaths are registered in the United Kingdom, and cause of death ascribed. What are the potential sources of error in routine mortality statistics?

4   Briefly describe some of the approaches that may be used to collect information for public health practice where routine sources of data on population characteristics, mortality, etc. do not exist.

5   Summarize some of the issues to be considered when comparing disease rates based on routine information sources over time or between places.

Now reflect again on what your skills and knowledge currently are, where there are gaps and any actions arising.

Public health standards	
Surveillance & assessment	
Promoting & protecting	
Developing quality & risk management	
Collaborative working for health	
Developing programmes & services & reducing inequalities	
Policy & strategy development & implementation	
Working with & for communities	
Strategic leadership	.
Research & Development	
Ethically managing self, people & resources	

3

Measuring the frequency of health problems

What are rates and why are they needed in public health?

What are incidence and prevalence and how are they related?

Why are standardized rates needed and how are they calculated?

After working through this chapter you should be able to:

- discuss the need for rates;
- explain what a rate is;
- define incidence and prevalence;
- describe the relationship between incidence and prevalence;
- describe what is meant by crude, specific and standardized rates;
- describe what is meant by crude, specific and standardized mortality rates;
- understand how directly and indirectly age-standardized rates are derived;
- appreciate the potential shortcomings of both indirect and direct methods of standardization.

Why are rates needed?

First, work through Exercise 3.1.

Exercise 3.1

Over the course of seven years 146 people were referred to a hospital plastic surgery unit because they had been bitten by a dog. Details of the breed of dog causing the bite were collected from 107 people. The main breeds responsible were as follows:

Staffordshire bull terrier	15 cases
Jack Russell	13 cases
Medium-sized mongrel	10 cases
Alsatian	9 cases
Labrador	8 cases
Collie	6 cases

Question: Does this mean that Staffordshire bull terriers are more likely to bite people than collies?

If your answer is 'No', or perhaps 'Not sure', what other information would you like before you could answer this question properly?

Source: Shewell, P. C. and Nancarrow, J.D. (1991) Dogs that bite, *British Medical Journal*, 303: 1512–13.

We hope you agree that it does not follow from the information in the first example that Staffordshire bull terriers are more likely to bite people than collies. Further information is required. Two pieces of information you may have thought of are, how many dogs are there in each breed, and how much time do those dogs spend around people? It is possible that collies are more likely to bite than Staffordshire bull terriers. This would be compatible with the results above if collies were much less commonly owned or spent less time with people. So to make a valid comparison we need to relate the number of bites for each breed to the number of dogs in that breed, or to the amount of time the dogs spend with people. In other words we need to use *rates*.

What is a rate?

In epidemiology a rate is a measure of how frequently an event occurs, in a defined population, over a specified period of time. All rates are ratios, which simply means that they consist of one number divided by another number. The top number is called the *numerator* and the bottom one the *denominator*. The numerator of a rate is the number of times the event of interest, such as a dog bite, occurs over a given time period. The denominator is usually the average population size (such as the population of dogs) over the same time period.

$$\text{Rate} = \frac{\text{Number of events in a specified time period}}{\text{Average population during the time period}}$$

The figure is usually multiplied by a convenient number to convert it from a fraction into a whole number. So for example, if multiplied by 1000, it would then be the number of events per 1000 population for the specified time period. Try comparing the rate of bites from collies and Staffordshire bull terriers in the town of Barking (Exercise 3.2).

Exercise 3.2

Here are some figures from the hypothetical town of Barking. In Barking, in 2005, 20 people were bitten by Staffordshire bull terriers and 15 people were bitten by collies. Barking has a dog registration scheme and, assuming that all dogs are registered, it is known that in 2005 the average population of Staffordshire bull terriers in Barking was 200, and of collies was 150. Two dog owners are having a fierce debate over which breed is more likely to bite people. Assuming that each breed of dog spends the same amount of time around people, settle the dispute by calculating biting rates for each breed in 2005.

You should have found that the biting rates for collies and Staffordshire bull terriers were the same, i.e., ten bites per 100 dogs per year.

What are incidence and prevalence?

You are likely to hear and read more about two types of rate than any others. They are called incidence and prevalence. These terms are used to refer to rates that measure the frequency of a disease or health condition in a population. The aim of this section is to explain what each term means, and how they differ. First, work through Exercise 3.3 (overleaf).

Exercise 3.3 may seem a little simple. It is supposed to. Many people find incidence and prevalence difficult concepts. In fact they are not, and you have just calculated the prevalence and incidence of the common cold among the hypothetical nursing home residents in the month of January.

Prevalence refers to *all* (prev*A*lence) people in a defined population with the disease or condition at a given point in time or over a given period of time. The general formula for calculating the prevalence rate is:

$$\text{Prevalence rate} = \frac{\text{Total number of cases in a specified time period}}{\text{Total number in the defined population}}$$

Exercise 3.3

A nursing home has 100 residents. On the first day in January ten residents had a cold. Over the month of January another 18 residents developed a cold. Assuming that the number of residents did not change over January, answer the following questions:

What proportion of the residents had a cold on the first day of January?

What proportion of the residents had a cold some time during the month of January?

What proportion of the residents who didn't have a cold at the start of January developed a cold during the month of January?

Point prevalence refers to the proportion of people in a population with a disease or condition at one point in time. The point prevalence of the common cold among the nursing home residents in Exercise 3.3 on the first day of January was 10 per cent (10/100). *Period prevalence* is the proportion of people in a population known to have or have had a disease or condition at any time during a specified time period. The period prevalence for the month of January of the common cold among the nursing home residents in Exercise 2.3 was 28 per cent (28/100).

Incidence differs from prevalence in that it refers only to *new* (iNcidence) cases of a disease or condition that develop in a population over a specified period of time. The general formula for the incidence rate is:

$$\text{Incidence} = \frac{\text{Number of new cases in specified time period}}{\text{Population at risk in this time period}}$$

The 'population at risk' is an important concept. It refers to all people who *could* become new cases. In Exercise 3.3, ten of the nursing home residents already had a cold at the start of January and so could not become a new case over that month. Hence 90 residents were 'at risk' of developing a cold for the first time during the month of January, and 18 did, giving an incidence of 20 per cent.

To consider the concept of 'population at risk' in more detail, work through Exercise 3.4.

Exercise 3.4

You are interested in the incidence of cancer of the uterus in your area. You find out the number of new cases over the past year from the cancer registry. This gives the numer- ator for calculating the incidence. The denominator is the population 'at risk'. Imagine you start with the number of the total population of your area for the last year. Make a list of everyone who should be excluded from this to leave you with the true population 'at risk'.

When calculating the incidence of cancer of the uterus you would clearly want to exclude men from the denominator. You would also want to exclude women who had had a hysterectomy, because without a uterus they can no longer be at risk. You would also want to exclude women who had already had cancer of the uterus diagnosed before the specified time period, and who therefore could not become a new case. In practice you might find it difficult to define the size of the population at risk accur- ately. For example, even if the total number of women is known with reasonable accuracy, information on the number of women with hysterectomies might be harder to find. By working through Exercise 3.4 it may also have struck you that it will often make sense to define the population at risk when calculating prevalence. For example, giving the prevalence of cancer of uterus for the total population (men and women) wouldn't make much sense because men cannot be affected by cancer of the uterus.

What is the relationship between incidence and prevalence?

The relationship between incidence and prevalence is summarized in the 'prevalence pot' (Figure 3.1). The amount of water in the pot represents how much of a particular disease there is in the population at any one time (the point prevalence). This is dependent on the rate of new cases of the disease entering the pot (the incidence) and the rate with which people with the disease leave the pot (recover, die, or leave the area) which is related to the duration of the disease. Notice that the prevalence pot in Figure 3.1 assumes that there is no migration of people with the disease into or out of the population.

A simple mathematical formula is often used to represent the relationship between incidence, prevalence and duration of a disease.

Prevalence = Incidence × Average duration of the disease

This formula is only valid in the 'steady state' (when incidence and average duration can be assumed to have been constant over a long period of time) in a population without migration, and when the prevalence of the disease is low (in other words, 10 per cent or less). None the less it is a useful summary of the relationships between incidence, prevalence and duration. Use the formula to solve the problems in Exercise 3.5.

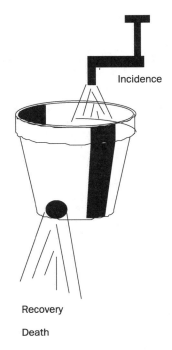

Incidence

Recovery

Death

Figure 3.1 The prevalence pot

Exercise 3.5

Use the formula:
 prevalence = incidence × average duration
 to fill in the empty boxes in the table below.

Condition	Incidence/100,000 population/year	Point prevalence/ 100,000 population	Average duration (years)
Epilepsy	30		13
Brain tumours	20	65	
Multiple sclerosis		60	12

Which is the commonest (most prevalent) condition?

Which condition has the shortest duration?

Answers: Epilepsy (390/100,000); brain tumours (3.25 year)

What is meant by crude, specific and standardized rates?

Rates can be presented as crude, specific or standardized. A *crude rate* is presented for an entire population. A *specific rate* is presented for a particular sub-group of a population. For example, age-specific rates are those presented for specified age groups in a population; and sex-specific for men and women separately. *Standardized rates* are used to compare two or more populations with the effects of differences in age or other confounding variables removed. For example, one would expect a population of predominantly young adults to have a much lower crude death rate than a population of predominantly old adults. Techniques of standardization can be used to compare these two populations with the effects of the age differences removed.

The uses of crude, specific and standardized rates are illustrated in the following sections on mortality rates.

Mortality rates

In Chapter 2 we noted that routine information sources on morbidity are very limited, but that information on mortality tends to be much more readily available. For this reason mortality rates are probably the single most important routinely available data source on the 'health' of populations. Familiarity with the use and interpretation of mortality rates is therefore very important.

Mortality rates are incidence rates – the incidence of death. In the rest of this section the uses and limitations of crude, specific, and standardized mortality rates are illustrated by comparing the mortality experience of two real populations in 2001. One population is that of England and Wales, and the other is from a demographic surveillance system in Tanzania, which was also used as an example in Chapter 2. In this system three contrasting areas of Tanzania are under surveillance, covering over 300,000 people, which is roughly 1 per cent of the total Tanzanian population. Regular censuses are used to count the number of residents by age and sex, and a system of key informants identifies deaths.

Crude mortality rates

The crude mortality rate for a given year can be defined as:

$$\frac{\text{all deaths during a the year}}{\text{population at the mid-year}}$$

Typically mortality statistics which are routinely available, are presented for a calendar year (i.e., January to December), and usually the rate is multiplied by 1000 to give the number of deaths per 1000 population per year.

Before you work through Exercise 3.6, think whether you expect that England and Wales or Tanzania will have the highest crude mortality rate?

Exercise 3.6

The table below shows the number of deaths, and mid-year populations for England and Wales and three surveillance sites combined in Tanzania in 2001. Complete the table by calculating the crude death rates.

	Total deaths	Mid-year population	Death rate per 1000 population per year
England and Wales	530,373	52,084,000	
Tanzanian sites	3625	345,935	

The crude death rates are very similar. Is this the answer you expected?

Does this mean, in your view, that the risk of death in these two populations is about the same?

If your answer to the above question is 'No', what reasons can you think of for the similarity in the crude rates?

Sources: Office of National Statistics, UK; Adult morbidity and mortality project, Ministry of Health, Tanzania.

Exercise 3.6 shows that the crude mortality rate in England and Wales is similar to that in Tanzania (i.e., 10.2 deaths per 1000 population per year versus 10.5 per 1000 per year). At first this result is surprising – one of the world's poorest countries has a similar crude mortality rate to one of the richest. Surely, mortality must be higher in Tanzania? The reason for this apparent paradox lies in the differences in age structure between the populations. This is addressed in the next section.

Age- and category-specific mortality rates

An age-specific mortality rate is simply the mortality rate for a particular age group. For example, the rate per 1000 for persons aged 45–54 would be:

$$\frac{\text{number of deaths in people aged 45–54}}{\text{mid-year population of 45–54 year olds}} \times 1000$$

Age-specific mortality rates for England and Wales and Tanzania are shown in Table 3.1. Notice that in every age group, apart from the two eldest, the rates are higher in Tanzania, often substantially so (particularly in the younger age groups) – yet the crude mortality rate is not very different. The reason for this that the age structures of the two populations are very different. A much larger proportion of the population in Tanzania consists of children and young adults. This is illustrated in Figure 3.2 which shows the distribution of the populations by broad age groups. Almost 60 per cent of the Tanzanian population is aged less than 25 years, compared to 30 per cent in England and Wales, whereas in England and Wales over 25 per cent of the population is aged 55 years or over, while in Tanzania it is around 10 per cent. You can see from Table 3.1 that although the age-specific rates in Tanzania tend to be higher than in England and Wales, the death rates in children and young adults

Table 3.1 Mortality rates by age group (men and women combined) in England and Wales (E&W) and Tanzania in 2001

Age group (years)	E&W deaths/1000	Tanzania deaths/1000	Rate ratio Tanzania/E&W
0–4	1.2	19.6	15.8
5–14	0.1	1.6	12.9
15–24	0.5	2.8	5.9
25–34	0.7	8.4	11.8
35–44	1.3	13.2	10.5
45–54	3.2	14.9	4.6
55–64	8.1	16.9	2.1
65–74	22.4	30.0	1.3
75–84	59.8	53.0	0.9
85+	164.0	149.7	0.9

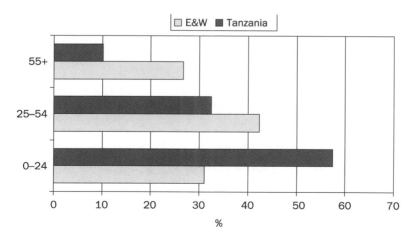

Figure 3.2 Percentage of the England and Wales and Tanzanian populations by broad age groups

(e.g., below 35 years) in Tanzania are still substantially lower than those in older people in England and Wales (e.g., 65 and above).

It is often informative to examine rates by other categories as well as age. For example, one could examine males and females separately. In most populations age-specific death rates are higher in men than in women.

Cause-specific mortality rates refer to rates from specific causes of death, such as lung cancer or heart disease. For example, the rate of death from heart disease in men aged 45–54 for one year would be computed as:

$$\frac{\text{Deaths from heart disease in men aged 45–54 in year}}{\text{Number of men aged 45–54 at mid-year}} \times 1000$$

Let's summarize this section. Crude mortality rates can be a very misleading way of comparing the mortality experience of different populations. Age is the single most important determinant of mortality and at the very least differences in age structure between the populations must be taken into account. Comparing age-specific death rates is one way to do this but can be cumbersome because it involves making many comparisons. However, single rates can be produced which have been adjusted for age differences between the populations. These are called age-adjusted or age-standardized rates.

How are age-standardized mortality rates produced?

Consider again the reason for a similar crude mortality rate in Tanzania to England and Wales, despite most of the age-specific rates being much higher in Tanzania. The reason is that in Tanzania a much larger proportion of the population is made up of children and young adults, and a much lower proportion is made up of older people, than in England and Wales. A crude mortality rate depends on the age-specific death rates *and* the proportion of the population in each of the age bands. This can be summarized in the following way:

Crude mortality rate = sum of (each age-specific mortality rate × proportion of the population in that age group)

There are two methods of age standardization: direct standardization and indirect standardization. The principle behind them both is the same.

In *direct standardization* the proportions in each age group of a *standard population* are applied to the age-specific death rates of the populations being compared. There are a small number of standard populations that are widely available. The World Health Organization, for example, produces a standard population based on the age distribution of the entire population of the world. This is called the world standard population, and it is based on the estimated average age distribution for the entire world from 2000 to 2025. This standard population has been used to calculate directly age-standardized death rates for England and Wales and for Tanzania, using the age-specific death rates in Table 3.1. The calculation is illustrated in Table 3.2.

Table 3.2 Calculation of directly age standardized death rates for England and Wales and Tanzania, using the world standard population, 2001

Age group (years)	Proportion of world standard population by age group	Proportion X age-specific death rate in E&W	Proportion X age-specific death rate in Tanzania
0–4	0.09	0.11	1.74
5–14	0.17	0.02	0.27
15–24	0.17	0.08	0.46
25–34	0.16	0.11	1.30
35–44	0.14	0.17	1.82
45–54	0.11	0.37	1.71
55–64	0.08	0.67	1.40
65–74	0.05	1.16	1.55
75–84	0.02	1.45	1.29
85+	0.01	1.04	0.95
Totals	1.00	5.19	12.50

The directly age-adjusted rate for England and Wales is 5.19 deaths per 1000 population per year, and for Tanzania it is 12.50. These can be shown as a ratio, one divided by the other (for example, 12.50/5.19 = 2.41). This is called a *standardized rate ratio* and indicates that when differences in age structure are taken into account, using the standard world population, death rates in Tanzania are 2.4 times higher than in England and Wales.

Indirect standardization follows the same principle as direct standardization but with one very important difference. In indirect standardization a standard population is used to provide age-specific death rates, rather than providing the proportions of the population in different age groups. The age-specific death rates of the standard population are applied to the age groups of the population to which it is being compared. This gives the number of deaths in each group that would be expected if the population had the same age-specific death rates as the standard population. Using the number of 'expected' deaths and the actual number of deaths observed, a figure called the standardized mortality ratio (SMR) can be calculated. This is derived as follows:

$$SMR = \frac{\text{Observed number of deaths}}{\text{Expected number of deaths}}$$

The figure is traditionally multiplied by 100 to avoid cumbersome fractions. If the standard population and the population being compared had the same mortality experience, then the figure would be 100 because the expected and observed number of deaths would be equal. An SMR of greater than 100 means that the mortality in the population being compared is higher than in the standard, and less than 100 means that the mortality is lower. Table 3.3 demonstrates the calculation of the 'expected' number of deaths for Tanzania using the age-specific death rates of England and Wales as standard.

Table 3.3 Calculation of the standardized mortality ratio for Tanzania using the age-specific death rates of England and Wales (from Table 3.1) as standard

Age group (years)	Population in the Tanzanian sites	'Expected' number of deaths based on age-specific death rates in E&W	Observed number of deaths
0–4	45,961	57.0	903
5–14	89,384	11.0	142
15–24	63,331	29.8	176
25–34	51,884	36.7	434
35–44	36,268	45.9	480
45–54	24,288	78.5	363
55–64	17,229	139.9	292
65–74	10,885	244.0	327
75–84	5128	306.6	272
85+	1577	258.6	236
Totals	345,935	1208.0	3625

Note: SMR (observed/expected deaths * 100) = 300.

Table 3.3 demonstrates that the SMR for Tanzania is 300. This means that there are 300 per cent more deaths (i.e., three times) more deaths in the Tanzanian population than would have occurred if it had the same the same age-specific death rates as England and Wales.

What are the potential shortcomings of age-standardized mortality rates?

There are two potential shortcomings of using age-standardized mortality rates to consider. The first is general and the second refers specifically to indirectly standardized rates.

First, using a single figure (the age-adjusted rate) inevitably hides the detail of the age-specific rates. Table 3.1 shows that in all the age groups below 55 years, the deaths rates in Tanzania are over four times higher, often markedly so, than in England and Wales. Above the age of 55 the death rates are much more similar between the two populations. The standardized rate ratio of 2.41 thus doesn't really reflect the situation in most of the age groups (it is closest to the situation in the 55 to 64-year age group), but provides an average figure across them all. The best way to give a clear picture of the situation is to describe the actual age-specific death rates.

The interpretation of one indirectly age-standardized rate, or SMR, is straight-forward. It is the comparison of the number of deaths that occurred with the number of deaths that would have occurred if the population had the same age-specific death rates as the standard population. Because SMRs are calculated by applying the age-specific death rates of the standard population to the age structure of the population of interest, they should not be used for comparing more than two populations, especially if those populations have different age structures.

Having noted that SMRs should only be used to compare the standard population and one other population, you need to be warned that you will often see SMRs used to compare several populations. If the population age structures are very different, as between England and Wales and Tanzania, then using SMRs is likely to be very misleading.

The reason that the indirect method of standardization remains popular is that it has two practical advantages over the direct method. The first is that you don't need to know the age-specific death rates of the population being compared. All you need are the total number of deaths (the observed deaths) and the age structure (to be able to calculate the expected deaths). The second advantage of the indirect method is that it is subject to less random error than the direct method. This is because in the direct method the number of deaths used to calculate the age-specific death rates will often be very small and subject to quite marked variation from year to year and between populations. By using only the total number of deaths (the observed deaths) the indirect method is less subject to this type of error.

Summary

1   Write a short paragraph to explain to a colleague why rates are needed to make comparisons between populations. (Try making up a hypothetical example of your own to illustrate the point.)

2   Give the general formula for a rate.

3   Give the general formulas for incidence and prevalence.

4   Describe the relationship between incidence, prevalence and disease duration.

5   Define the following terms:
    • crude mortality rate
    • age-specific mortality rate
    • disease-specific mortality rate

6   Describe the differences between direct and indirect age standardization.

7   Explain why the use of indirect standardization to compare more than two populations could in some circumstances be misleading.

Now reflect again on what your skills and knowledge currently are, where there are gaps and any actions arising.

Public health standards	
Surveillance & assessment	
Promoting & protecting	
Developing quality & risk management	
Collaborative working for health	
Developing programmes & services & reducing inequalities	
Policy & strategy development & implementation	
Working with & for communities	
Strategic leadership	
Research & Development	
Ethically managing self, people & resources	

4

Measures of risk

What are the definitions of hazard and risk?

What is a relative risk?

What is a risk factor?

What is the definition of attributable risk?

How do attributable and relative risk differ?

After working through this chapter you should be able to:

- define the terms 'hazard' and 'risk' as used in epidemiology;
- define relative risk;
- define and discuss what is meant by the term 'risk factor';
- define the terms attributable risk (exposed) and attributable risk (population);
- describe the main assumptions on which the use of attributable risk is based;
- discuss the relevance to public health of relative risk and attributable risk (exposed and population).

What are hazard and risk?

Hazard and risk are terms used in everyday language. However, in epidemiology they have quite specific meanings. Hazard refers to the potential to cause harm, whereas risk refers to the likelihood of causing harm. You can think of the difference between a domestic cat and a lion. The lion is a much greater hazard (it has more potential to cause harm – unless you are allergic to cat hair). However, if the lion is safely in a cage or in an environment where it cannot attack humans, the likelihood of harm may be very low. To take a risk can mean to undertake a dangerous activity. Rock climbing or hang gliding are often described as risky activities. To take a risk also implies chance: that there is a chance of an unpleasant or damaging event occurring.

Uses of the term risk from everyday language also help to capture the meaning of the term risk in epidemiology. It is about the chance or probability of events occurring. In epidemiology, as in everyday use, the events are usually undesirable, such as deaths or episodes of disease. However, a definition of risk that fits its use in epidemiology is simply this: *the probability that an event will occur*. The event need not be undesirable. It would make sense, for example, to refer to the risk (or probability) of cure of a disease by a particular drug.

Concepts of risk, or the probability of events, are central to epidemiology. This chapter aims to illustrate the basic concepts. All the examples in this chapter are based on a landmark study of modern epidemiology. It is a study of the relationship between smoking and cause of death in British doctors. You have already come across data from this study in Chapter 1. The references for the papers on which these examples are based are given below in Exercise 4.1 and you may find it helpful to look them up. Work through this exercise now.

Exercise 4.1

In October 1951 a short questionnaire was sent to the 59,600 men and women whose names were on the Medical Register of the United Kingdom. The questionnaire sought information on the smoking habits of the doctors. 40,637 (68%) doctors returned completed questionnaires. The number of doctors who had died, and their causes of death, were obtained – mainly from death certificates. Between the 1st of November 1951 and the 31st of October 1961 there were 4963 deaths. The death rates by smoking status for different causes of death are shown in the table below.

	Deaths per 1000 persons per year			
Cause of death	*Total population*	*Non-smokers*	*All cigarette smokers*	*Cigarette smokers of >25 a day*
All causes	14.05	12.06	16.32	19.67
Lung cancer	0.65	0.07	1.20	2.23
Coronary heart disease	3.99	3.31	4.57	4.97

What are the risks of death in the non-smokers and those smoking 25 or more cigarettes a day?

What is the risk of death from lung cancer in non-smokers, and the risk of death from lung cancer in those smoking 25 or more cigarettes a day?

Can you conclude from the figures in the table that smoking increases the risk of death?

Source: Doll, R. and Hill, A.B. (1964) Mortality in relation to smoking: ten years' observation of British doctors, *British Medical Journal*, June, pp. 1399–410, 1460–7.

The risks of death in Exercise 4.1 are in fact the death rates. So the risk of death (from all causes) for non-smokers was 12.06 per 1000 persons per year, and for heavy smokers (25 or more cigarettes a day) was 19.67 per 1000 persons per year. If you wished, you could express these as per centages, i.e., 1.206 per cent per year and 1.967 per cent per year respectively. These figures represent the *absolute risk* of death among the non-smokers and heavy smokers in this study. Absolute risk is the same as the incidence rate, in this case the incidence of death.

You may feel that the figures in the table provide strong evidence that smoking increases the risk (or incidence) of death. However, you may also feel that more information is required. At the very least you would want to know that the smokers and non-smokers were of similar ages – if the smokers were older, then of course they would have higher death rates because the risk of death increases with age. In fact the figures in the table in Exercise 3.1 have been directly standardized (the technique is described in Chapter 2) to take account of differences in age and sex composition between the smokers and non-smokers. Of course, there may still be other differences between the smokers and non-smokers which account for the difference in the risk of death. The issue of deciding if a factor causes a disease is discussed in more detail in Chapter 6.

What is relative risk?

Relative risk is used to compare the incidence of a disease or condition between a group with a particular attribute or exposure to one without. It has the following form:

$$\frac{\text{Incidence in group with attribute or exposure}}{\text{Incidence in group without attribute or exposure}}$$

This is illustrated in Exercise 4.2. Work through this now.

Exercise 4.2

Taking the figures from the table in Exercise 4.1, the relative risk of all those smoking for death from lung cancer is:

$$\frac{1.20}{0.07} = 17.1$$

In plain English this means that those smoking were 17 times more likely to die from lung cancer than non-smokers.

The relative risk of death from lung cancer for heavy smokers compared to non-smokers is:

$$\frac{2.23}{0.07} = 31.9$$

Now calculate the relative risks of death from coronary heart disease for smokers compared to non-smokers and heavy smokers compared to non-smokers.

Answers: $4.57/3.31 = 1.4$, and $4.97/3.31 = 1.5$.

Relative risk is a measure of the strength of an association between an exposure or attribute and a disease. If the relative risk is 1, then the incidence in the two groups is the same. If it is greater than 1, then the attribute or exposure is associated with an increased incidence of the disease, and if less than 1, with a decreased incidence of the disease. For example, in the study of British doctors and smoking, there was clearly a very strong association between mortality from lung cancer and smoking (relative risk 17.1) but a much less strong relationship between mortality from coronary heart disease and smoking (relative risk 1.4). An exposure which is positively associated with the occurrence of a disease, such as smoking is with lung cancer, is often called a risk factor for that disease.

What is the meaning of the term 'risk factor'?

The idea that different exposures, behaviours and personal attributes influence our risk of developing disease is a very old idea. The concept of 'risk factors', however, comes from modern epidemiology. It has its origins in some of the large prospective epidemiological studies (studies in which people are followed up over time to see who develops a disease and who doesn't) that were started after the Second World War. The study of the association of smoking behaviour of British doctors with causes of death is an example of this type of study. Another famous study which helped to establish the concept of 'risk factor' began in a small town in New England in the United States of America. The town is called Framingham and in the late 1940s male and female residents aged 30 to 59 years underwent physical examinations, answered questions on personal behaviours such as smoking, and had blood tests. Over 5000 who were free of coronary heart disease at the time of the examination were re-examined several times over many years to determine who had developed coronary heart disease. In this way it was discovered that an increased risk of developing coronary heart disease was associated with smoking, high blood pressure, high serum cholesterol and other factors. These factors were called 'risk factors' for coronary heart disease.

The whole aim of identifying risk factors for a disease is to try and identify factors which may be causes of the disease and which, if removed or modified, would prevent the disease occurring. However, there is one very important message to take away from this section of the chapter. When an exposure or attribute is identified as a risk factor for a disease, it simply means that *it is associated with an increased probability (risk) of the disease occurring. It does not mean that the factor is a cause of the disease.* For example, epidemiological studies have identified well over 200 risk factors for coronary heart disease. These include not having siestas, snoring, having English as a mother tongue and not eating mackerel. These factors have been associated with an increased risk of the disease but they do not indicate that they are causal. Changing the mother tongue in Britain to Italian is unlikely by itself to lower the levels of heart disease! Some authors have suggested that the term risk factor should be dropped and replaced by risk marker or risk indicator. These latter terms better convey the fact it is a statistical association between the exposure or attribute and the outcome and not necessarily a causal relationship. These issues are considered further in Chapter 6.

What is attributable risk?

Attributable risk is used to provide an assessment of how much of a disease is 'due to' an exposure and so how much *might* be prevented if an exposure is removed.

Definitions of two types of attributable risk are given below. The first is for how much a disease among the *exposed* is 'due to' the exposure. The second is how much of the disease among the *total population* is 'due to' the exposure.

- *Attributable risk (exposed)* is the rate of a disease or condition among exposed individuals that can be attributed to the exposure.
- *Attributable risk (population)* is the rate of a disease or condition among the total population which can be attributed to the exposure.

The general formulae for calculating attributable risk exposed and population are as follows.

Attributable risk (exposed) = Incidence among the exposed – incidence among non-exposed

Attributable risk (population) = Incidence among total population – incidence among non-exposed

These are often presented as proportions. For example the per centage of cases of a disease in a population that are attributable to an exposure is:

$$\frac{\text{Incidence among total population} - \text{incidence among non-exposed}}{\text{Incidence among total population}} \times 100$$

By working through Exercise 4.3 (overleaf) you'll get a better idea of how attributable risk is calculated and what it means.

How should attributable risk be interpreted?

The simplest interpretation of attributable risk is that it represents the amount of the occurrence of a disease which is due to a particular exposure. So, for example, in the study of smoking among British doctors, smoking 'caused' 0.58 deaths from lung cancer per 1000 population per year, representing 89 per cent of all deaths from lung cancer (see Exercise 4.3). This interpretation, however, depends on two assumptions. The first is that the exposure (in this case smoking) causes the disease (lung cancer). The second is that other causes of the disease are equally distributed among the exposed (smokers) and unexposed (non-smokers).

A further interpretation that is usually placed upon attributable risk is that it represents the amount of a disease that could be prevented if the exposure were removed. This interpretation is based on a further assumption: that the rate of the disease in the exposed group will return to that in the non-exposed if the exposure is

Exercise 4.3

Look through the calculations of attributable risk (exposed) and attributable risk (population) for smoking and lung cancer. The figures are taken from the table in example 4.2.

Attributable risk (exposed) = 1.20 − 0.07 = 1.13 per 1000 persons per year

This can be interpreted as meaning that out of the 1.2 deaths from lung cancer per 1000 persons per year among the smokers, 1.13 were due to smoking. This can be expressed as a proportion, i.e.:

$$\frac{1.20 - 0.07}{1.20} \times 100 = 94\%$$

This can be interpreted as meaning that 94 percent of the deaths from lung cancer among the smokers were due to smoking.

Attributable risk (population) = 0.65 − 0.07 = 0.58 per 1000 persons per year

This can be interpreted as meaning that in the total population 0.58 per 1000 deaths per year from lung cancer were due to smoking, or put as a proportion (0.58/0.65 × 100), 89% of the lung cancer deaths in the total population were due to smoking.

Using the figures in the table in Exercise 4.1, carry out the same calculations for deaths from coronary heart disease.

Answers: AR (exposed) 1.26/1000/yr, 28%; AR (population) 0.68/1000/yr, 17%.

removed. How good this assumption is will depend on the exposure and disease. In the study of British doctors, for example, the death rates from lung cancer in those who had given up smoking did fall, but only in those who had given up smoking for around 20 years did the death rates approach those of non-smokers.

Let's summarize this section. Attributable risk is usually interpreted as providing an estimate of how much of a disease could be prevented if a particular exposure were removed. This interpretation is based on three assumptions: that the exposure causes the disease; that other factors causing the disease are equally distributed between the exposed and non-exposed groups; and that the rates of disease in the exposed group would fall to the rates in the non-exposed when the exposure were removed. Because of these assumptions, attributable risk is best regarded as providing an assessment of the *maximum possible benefit* of removing the exposure.

What is the relevance to public health of relative risk and attributable risk?

Relative risk and attributable risk provide two very different types of information. Relative risk is a measure of the strength of the association between an exposure and a disease. It is used to help assess whether or not an exposure is one of the causes of a disease. The strength of the association and whether or not there is a 'dose response' relationship between the occurrence of the disease and the exposure are two factors often used to assess if the exposure is likely to be causal. The strong association between smoking and lung cancer and the fact that the more cigarettes smoked, the stronger the association (e.g., see Exercise 4.2: the relative risk for heavy smokers was 31.9 and for all smokers 17.1) are two factors which, together with others, have led to the conclusion that smoking causes lung cancer.

The attributable risk (population) provides an estimate of the benefit that might be expected within the total population if exposure to a given factor is removed. Thus attributable risk (population) is helpful when guiding preventive health measures aimed at improving the health of a population. The potential benefits of removing different exposures can be assessed using attributable risk. This can be useful in helping to decide which exposures it is worth trying to prevent.

Finally, it is worth appreciating that the magnitude of the relative risk does not indicate the magnitude of the attributable risk. You can see this by looking again at Exercise 4.3. Both the attributable risk (exposed) and attributable risk (population) are higher for smoking and coronary heart disease than they are for smoking and lung cancer. This implies that if smoking were prevented in this population, more deaths would be prevented from coronary heart disease than from lung cancer. This is simply due to the fact that coronary heart disease is a much commoner cause of death than lung cancer. Look again at the table in Exercise 4.1. The death rate in the total population from coronary heart disease was 3.99/1000 compared to 0.65/1000 for lung cancer. Seventeen per cent (the proportion of coronary heart disease deaths in the total population 'due to' smoking) of 3.99 is greater than 89 per cent (the proportion of lung cancer deaths in the total population 'due to' smoking) of 0.65.

Summary

1   Describe what are meant by the terms 'hazard' and 'risk' as used in epidemiology.

2   Give the general formula for relative risk.

3   A lay person has read of 200 'risk factors' for coronary heart disease. S/he is confused and worried about what it all means. Write a short paragraph to reassure him/her and explain what a 'risk factor' is.

4   Give the general formulae for attributable risk (exposed) and attributable risk (population).

5   Attributable risk is often interpreted as giving the amount of a disease that would be prevented if the exposure were removed. What are the assumptions on which this interpretation is based?

6   Write a short paragraph contrasting the different uses in public health of relative risk and attributable risk.

Now reflect again on what your skills and knowledge currently are, where there are gaps and any actions arising.

Public health standards	
Surveillance & assessment	
Promoting & protecting	
Developing quality & risk management	
Collaborative working for health	
Developing programmes & services & reducing inequalities	
Policy & strategy development & implementation	
Working with & for communities	
Strategic leadership	
Research & Development	
Ethically managing self, people & resources	

5

Epidemiological study designs

What types of epidemiological study are there?

Which study designs are used to identify the amount of a disease or health condition?

Which study designs are used to identify possible causes of a disease or health condition?

By working through this chapter you should be able to:

- provide a simple classification of the different types of study;
- describe and give examples of the main uses of each type of epidemiological study;
- discuss the strengths and weaknesses of the different types of epidemiological study designs.

What types of epidemiogical study are there?

There is no single agreed classification of epidemiological studies, and in your reading you are likely to come across different terms for the same type of study. One approach to their classification is to consider their role within public health. A broad definition of public health, referred to in Chapter 1, is, 'collective action for sustained population-wide health improvement'. Epidemiology is one of the core scientific disciplines that provides information which is essential (but by itself not enough) to guide and monitor public health activity. In Chapter 1, epidemiology was defined as, 'the study of the distribution and determinants of health-related states or events in human populations and the application of this study to the control of health problems'.

Generally epidemiological studies are used to provide information on three areas:

- on the *distribution and frequency* of diseases, and on the frequency and distribution of known and possible causes of diseases in populations – such studies are usually called *descriptive*;
- on the strength of *associations* between diseases and other factors (such as smoking, diet or socio-economic status), with particular emphasis on whether such associations are causal – such studies are usually called *analytical*;
- on whether *interventions* aimed at preventing a disease or improving its outcome actually do so – such studies are usually called *intervention* studies.

Within these three broad categories several types of study can be identified. These are summarized in Table 5.1.

Table 5.1 A classification of the main types of epidemiological studies

Main category	Types within category
Descriptive studies	Descriptions based on data sources already available. Cross-sectional (prevalence) surveys.
Analytical studies	Ecological. Cross-sectional. Case-control. Cohort.
Intervention studies	Clinical trial. Community trial.

What are descriptive studies used for and what types are there?

Uses of descriptive studies

Descriptive studies are used to provide information on the frequency of health states and their known and possible causes by person, place and time. Such information is crucial to guide the planning of health promotion and disease prevention activities, to guide the planning of health services and may also provide important clues as to the causes of different health states. Some of the factors to consider under the headings of person, place and time are outlined below.

Person – e.g., for a certain health state, how old are the people who get it?, what sex are they?, what is their socio-economic status?, what is their occupation?, what is their ethnic group?, what are their lifestyles?, such as smoking and diet, and so on?

Place – e.g., is the occurrence of the health state more frequent in some geographical areas than others, such as between countries, areas within countries or areas within cities?; do members of an ethnic group who have a low rate of the disease in one area also have a low rate when members of that ethnic group move to another area, and so on?

Time – e.g., has the frequency of the health state changed over long periods of time, such as several years?; does the frequency of the disease vary throughout the year, and so on?

Descriptive studies based on routinely available data sources

Many descriptive studies can be carried out using the type of routine information described in Chapter 2. A classic example of how thought-provoking simple descriptive data can be was shown in Chapter 1, Exercise 1.4. This exercise demonstrated that most of the fall in deaths from TB in England and Wales during the nineteenth and twentieth centuries occurred before effective drug therapy or BCG vaccination was available. Exercise 5.1 is also based on routinely collected mortality data in England

---

Exercise 5.1

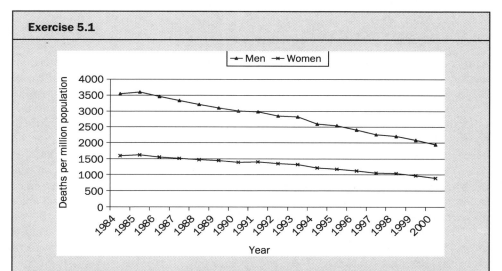

Age-standardized death rates from ischaemic heart disease in England and Wales

The graph shows trends in death rates from ischaemic heart disease per million population in men and women in England and Wales. Both the male and female rates have been age-standardized to the same population (the European standard), allowing comparison to be made between them and over time despite any differences in age structure (see Chapter 4 for an explanation of age standardization).

What possible explanations can you think of for:

1.   The downward trends in death rates?

2.   The differences in rates between men and women?

Source: Office of National Statistics, UK.

and Wales. It shows age-standardized death rates from ischaemic heart disease in men and women in England and Wales between 1984 and 2000. Look at this now.

The data in Exercise 5.1 shows how thought-provoking basic descriptive data can be. First, there is the very big difference in death rates in coronary heart disease between men and women. The reasons for this difference remain open to some debate and continuing research. They include the possible impact of biological differences, such as in sex hormone levels, on ischaemic heart disease incidence, as well as differences in behaviours between men and women, such as in smoking, diet and approaches to dealing with stress. The downward trends are intriguing, and have been seen in most industrialized countries. In-depth analyses to assess the reasons for these trends in several countries have suggested that improvements in both risk factors (e.g., lower levels of smoking, blood pressure and blood cholesterol), and in medical care (e.g., through new drugs and other advances) have played major roles.

Cross-sectional (prevalence) surveys

As discussed in Chapter 2, routinely available data tend to be very limited. Determining the frequency of a particular health state or disease often requires a special study, the most common type being what is called a cross-sectional or prevalence survey. In a *cross-sectional* survey the health status individuals in a defined population, and any other factors of interest, are measured at one point in time. The most important use of cross-sectional surveys is to find out the proportion of people within a population who have a particular disease (or any other condition) of interest. Therefore another commonly applied name for cross-sectional surveys is *prevalence* surveys. Knowing the prevalence of conditions is often an essential first step to be able to plan public health activities to tackle them. Exercise 5.2 uses a prevalence survey from two areas of Tanzania as an example. Have a look at this now.

Exercise 5.2 helps to highlight some of the issues to consider in the interpretation of prevalence studies. They include whether simply by chance unrepresentative samples of households could have been chosen and thus give a false impression of the picture in the underlying population. In general, the smaller the sample size, the greater is this possibility. In the study in Exercise 5.2 nearly 1000 adults in each area were examined, making this a very unlikely explanation for the differences. However, another area to consider is what proportion of those who were invited to take part actually agreed to take part in the survey, and were those who participated systematically different from those who didn't (thus giving a biased picture)? In Exercise 5.2 almost 90 per cent of those in Hai participated, and around 65 per cent in Dar es Salaam. Although it seems unlikely, it needs to be asked whether those who participated in Dar es Salaam were more likely to have diabetes than those who didn't participate, thus giving a falsely high prevalence. Another problem you may have considered is in the measurement of fasting glucose. For example, were all the participants fasting, and, if not, is it possible that fewer were fasting in Dar es Salaam, thus tending to inflate the differences between the areas? Having considered these and other issues the authors concluded that there was a real and substantial difference in the prevalence of diabetes between these two areas. The next chapter addresses in more detail the interpretation of the findings of epidemiological studies.

Exercise 5.2

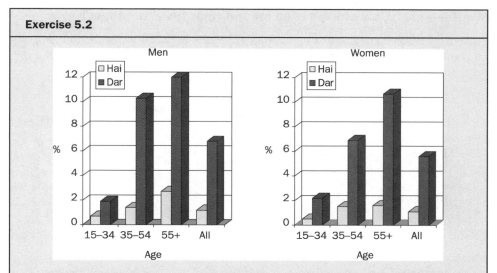

Prevalence (%) of diabetes in men and women in a rural (Hai) and urban (Dar) area of Tanzania

The graphs show the prevalence (%) of diabetes in men and women in a rural and urban part of Tanzania. These graphs are based on figures from a survey in which households were selected at random in a village in Hai district and in an area of Dar es Salaam. All adults aged 15 years and over were invited to participate. Each participant was asked to fast over night and had their blood glucose measured on a finger prick sample the next morning. They were also asked if they had ever been told that they had diabetes, and if so by whom and how the diagnosis was made. All those whose blood result was higher than the World Health Organization diagnostic level (7.0 mmol/l for fasting plasma glucose) or reported a diagnosis from a medical practitioner were counted as having diabetes.

The prevalence of diabetes clearly appears to be much higher in the urban area.

Before accepting this conclusion, what else would you like to know about the study and how it was conducted?

Source: Aspray et al. (2000) *Transactions of the Royal Society of Tropical Medicine & Hygiene*, 94: 637–44.

Prevalence surveys may also be used to examine associations between a disease and possible causes of the disease. Thus, depending on how they are analysed and used, cross-sectional studies can be classified with either descriptive or analytical studies. The use of cross-sectional studies to examine associations between diseases and possible causes is discussed in the next section.

What are analytical studies used for and what types are there?

Analytical studies are used to identify associations between a disease and possible causes of the disease. Types of study which are used for this are ecological, cross-sectional, cohort and case-control studies (Figure 5.1).

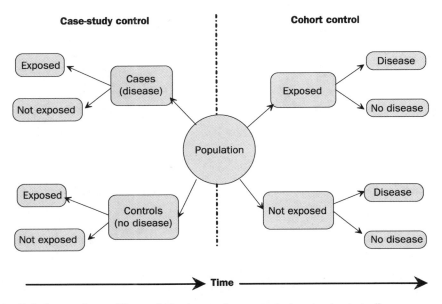

Figure 5.1 Comparison of the main features of case-control and cohort studies

Ecological studies

In an ecological study, data is collected on whole groups or populations of people rather than on individuals. Usually routinely collected data on disease rates are compared with data on the possible causes of the disease within the same populations or groups. Exercise 5.3 is based on some results from a landmark study in the United States that examined the relationship between the prevalence of dental carries within a population and the concentration of fluoride in the water supply. Have a look at this exercise now.

The main advantage of ecological studies is that they tend to be conducted using routinely collected data and therefore they can usually be done quickly and inexpensively. The study in Exercise 5.3 suggested that towns with higher fluoride levels in the water have lower levels of caries. The major disadvantage of ecological studies is that they are based on groups of people and not on individuals. It is possible there are many other differences between the towns in Exercise 5.3 apart from fluoride level which might account for the different levels of caries: an association found at the group level may not exist at the individual level, or conversely there may be no association found at the group level when in fact one does exist at the individual level. In either case

Exercise 5.3

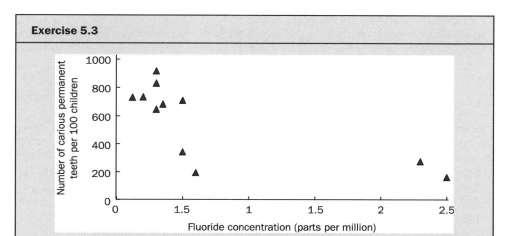

Relationship between prevalence of dental caries and water fluoride concentration

The graph shows the relationship between the number of dental caries per 100 children (aged 12 to 14 years) and the concentration of fluoride in the water supply for 11 towns in the United States.

What is the nature of the relationship?

What explanations can you think of for this relationship?

Source: Dean, T. (1938) Endemic Fluorosis and its relation to dental caries, *Public Health Reports*, 53(33): 1443–52.

the wrong conclusion would be drawn from the ecological study. This type of misleading result is called an 'ecological fallacy'. Therefore ecological studies are best seen as useful means of generating hypotheses on the possible determinants of health states, hypotheses which can be tested in more detailed studies, which, of course, was the case with the hypothesis that fluoride helps to protect against tooth decay.

Cross-sectional studies

As was discussed in the previous section, cross-sectional studies or prevalence surveys may be used to identify associations between diseases and possible causes. For example, in the study shown in Exercise 5.2 there was found to be a strong association between being overweight or obese and the presence of diabetes. Indeed, in this study it was estimated that at least 60 per cent of the difference in diabetes prevalence between the rural and urban area could be due to differences in overweight and obesity between those areas. However, the drawback of a prevalence survey for examining associations is that the study is only at one point in time. Thus, whether obesity leads to diabetes, or whether diabetes leads to obesity cannot be determined from this type of study. Given such an observation, one might hypothesize that obesity increases the risk of developing diabetes and then undertake more appropriate studies to see if the hypothesis is correct. There are, however, some situations in which one can be confident that the risk marker preceded the onset of the disease. For example, genetically determined factors such as sex and blood group clearly must precede the onset of any disease developed in later life, but even in this situation the fact that there is an association doesn't mean that it is the cause of the disease. Assessing whether an association is likely to be causal is covered in Chapter 6. Looking for associations within cross-sectional studies is best seen as an aid to generating ideas on the causes of a disease or other health condition: if associations are found, this can provide the basis for more detailed work to try and determine if such associations are causal.

Case-control studies

Case-control studies compare people with the disease of interest (cases) to people without the disease (controls) and look for differences in past exposure to possible causes of the disease. A well-known example of a case-control study is shown in Exercise 1.5, in Chapter 1. The study was investigating the possible causes of cancer of the lung. Cases (people with lung cancer) and controls (people without lung cancer) were both asked about their past exposure to a variety of possible causes, one of which was tobacco smoke. It was found that controls were more likely to have been light or non-smokers, and cases more likely to have been heavy smokers. This was one of the first studies to strongly suggest the link between smoking and lung cancer. Exercise 5.4 provides another example of a case-control study. It is based on a hypothetical food poisoning outbreak. Case-control studies are very commonly used in this situation to try and identify which food was responsible. Look at this now.

The figures in Exercise 5.4 provide strong evidence that the salmon mousse was the source of the food poisoning, but there are other possible explanations. For example, people who ate the mousse may have been more likely to eat another dish as well, perhaps it was served with a sauce which was the cause of the food poisoning. This is an example of confounding, where another variable is associated with both the exposure of interest (in this case eating salmon mousse), and the outcome (vomiting). The importance of considering confounding in investigating the association between two variables is discussed further in Chapter 6. This might then explain why not all the cases reported eating mousse, maybe they tried the sauce only. However, also note in Exercise 5.4 that food poisoning was simply referred to as people who reported vomiting, and not all the vomiting may have been due to food poisoning. Conversely, the 16 people who ate the mousse but didn't vomit may have had other symptoms of food poisoning or may not have eaten enough to become ill.

In case-control studies the strength of the association between a health state and an exposure is measured by calculating the odds ratio. This is illustrated in Exercise 5.4. As discussed in Chapter 4, relative risk provides the most direct measure of an association between a disease and possible causes. Relative risk is the incidence of

Exercise 5.4

The table below shows some hypothetical results from an investigation of a food poisoning outbreak at a wedding reception. There were 100 guests and 25 reported vomiting within 24 hours of attending the reception. A list was made of all the foods available at the reception and all the guests were asked which they had eaten. The table shows the results for the salmon mousse.

	Ate salmon mousse	
Food poisoning	Yes	No
Yes	20	5
No	15	60

The strength of association between having food poisoning and eating the salmon mousse is calculated as the 'odds ratio' (OR for short), which is the chance of eating the mousse (exposure) among those with food poisoning (20/5) divided by the chance of exposure in those without food poisoning (15/60), which works out at 16. Thus in this hypothetical example, those with food poisoning were 16 times more likely to report eating salmon mousse than those without.

Does this mean salmon mousse was the source of the food poisoning?

If it does, what explanation might there be for the five cases who said they didn't eat mousse, and the 15 who didn't report vomiting who said they did eat the mousse?

the disease in individuals exposed to a potential cause divided by the incidence of the disease in the unexposed. Case-control studies start with people with and without the disease of interest and do not therefore measure disease incidence. However, it can be shown that if certain conditions are met, the odds ratio found in a case-control study is a valid and close estimate of relative risk. These conditions are not discussed in detail here, but include that the cases of the disease are newly diagnosed (that they are what are called 'incident cases'), that prevalent cases are not included in the control group, and that the selection of cases and controls is independent of exposure status. Most case-control studies are designed to meet these conditions, and it is a big bonus of the case-control study design that it is able to provide a valid estimate of relative risk.

In mischievous moments, some commentators have suggested that the results from case-control studies must always be taken with a pinch of salt. This is because case-control studies are particularly prone to some types of bias. Bias, which can be defined as systematic error or deviation of results or inferences from the truth, is discussed in more detail in the next chapter. Two types of bias to which case-control studies are particularly prone are touched on here. The first is information bias, that is bias arising from the way information is collected in the study. Case-control studies are particularly prone to one type of information bias, known as recall bias. Recall bias refers to differences between cases and controls in the completeness of recall to memory of past events or experiences. This may arise because cases try harder to remember past events than controls – the presence of a serious disease can certainly focus the mind, and lead the subject to search their memory for events which may provide some explanation as to why they developed the disease. Recall bias may also arise because the person interviewing the cases and controls questions the cases more thoroughly than the controls. The interviewer may well have his/her own views about the causes of the disease and so tend to press the cases a little harder on these issues than the controls. Another form of bias to which case-control studies are particularly prone arises from the selection and comparison of cases and controls. It needs to be crystal clear what population the cases in the study represent. The controls should be representative of the population from which the cases came, which is generally taken to mean that had the controls developed the disease, they would have been selected as cases in the study.

Case-control studies have several advantages. They are comparatively cheap and quick to conduct, giving an answer as to the possible causes of a disease within a relatively short period of time. Because the investigator starts with people with a given health condition, rather than following people up to see who will develop the disease as in cohort studies (described below), they are good for investigating the causes of rare diseases. In addition a whole range of possible causes for a single disease can be investigated within one study.

Cohort studies

In a cohort study two or more groups of people who are free of the disease or other health condition of interest, but who differ according to exposure to a potential cause or causes, are followed up over time to compare the incidence of the health condition in each group. (The term *cohort* simply refers to any designated group of people who are followed up over a period of time.) The study of doctors and smoking, described in Exercise 4.1 of Chapter 4, is an example of a cohort study. This study was set up after the case-control study, described in Exercise 1.5 in Chapter 1, that compared patients with lung cancer to patients with other conditions (mainly patients with cancers at other sites) and suggested the link between smoking and lung cancer. It is quite common for a cohort study to be set up to determine if associations found in a case-control study are also found in a cohort study. If the associations are found in both types of study, this strengthens the evidence that the associations are real. Whether or not the associations are *causal* is a separate question and addressed in detail in the next chapter.

In cohort studies the strength of the association between the disease (or other outcome of interest) and possible cause of the disease is measured by comparing the incidence of the disease in those exposed to the possible cause and the incidence of the disease in those not exposed.

Because in cohort studies exposures to potential causes of a disease are defined before the disease develops, they are less prone to information bias than case-control studies. In addition, cohort studies directly measure the relative risks associated with different exposures. For these reasons in particular, the information derived from cohort studies is often given greater weight than information derived from case-control studies. Cohort studies are also good for looking at the effects of rare exposures, because individuals can be selected on the basis of exposure at the start of the study. A cohort study can also examine multiple possible outcomes from a single exposure.

However, cohort studies do have several drawbacks. They are a very inefficient way of looking for the potential causes of rare diseases. For example, in a disease with an incidence of one per 100,000 per year, around one million individuals would need to be followed up for ten years to collect 100 cases. It is important that as many as possible of the individuals who originally entered the study are followed up. Keeping track of individuals is often an expensive and time-consuming process, but if losses to follow up are large, the findings may be quite misleading (because those lost to follow up may differ from the rest). Finally cohort studies (unless a 'historical cohort study' – described below) do not give quick answers. Often follow up over several years is required to collect enough cases of the disease to allow meaningful analysis.

Cohort and case-control studies can be regarded as investigating the potential causes of a disease from opposite directions. In a cohort study one starts with people free from the disease but exposed to different potential causes of the disease. In a case-control study one starts with people with and without the disease and then assesses their past exposure to potential causes of the disease. The relationship between cohort and case-control studies is illustrated in Figure 5.1. Because case-control studies look back in time, they are often called *retrospective studies*; and because cohort studies normally follow people up over time they are often called *prospective studies*. However, these names can be confusing and are best avoided. For example, it is possible to have a 'retrospective' or 'historical' cohort study, in which the exposure status of individuals is identified from previous medical records and the individuals are then examined to determine their current health status. The key point is not whether the investigation is retrospective or prospective, but whether the starting point was to identify individuals with or without a particular health condition (case-control study) or to identify individuals according to their exposure status and free of the disease or health condition (cohort study).

Nested case-control studies

A neat and increasingly used study design which combines some of the advantages of the cohort and case-control approaches is called the *nested case-control study*. In this design, data on exposure status are collected on a cohort of individuals, and thus following the cohort study approach exposure status is defined prior to the development of the health condition or disease of interest. This cohort is followed up and people who develop the disease of interest identified. Rather than comparing them with *all* the individuals who do not develop the disease, controls, perhaps two or three per case, are selected from the cohort and the study is then carried out like a case-control study. This makes the study much cheaper and quicker to carry out. This is particularly useful if the measurements of the exposure are expensive. For example, blood samples on every member of the cohort could be taken at the outset of the study and stored in a freezer. Only those samples of people who develop the disease (cases) and those chosen as controls will then be analysed.

What are intervention studies used for and what types are there?

The key difference between analytical and intervention studies is this: in an analytical study the investigator simply observes the exposure status of individuals; in an intervention study the investigator intervenes to change the exposure status of individuals to determine what happens when this is done. In short, the investigator is conducting an experiment and for this reason another name for intervention studies is 'experimental studies'.

There are two broad types of intervention study: clinical trials and community trials. These study types are analogous to two types of analytical studies: cohort and ecological studies respectively. In a clinical trial the unit of study is the individual and the investigator intervenes to change the exposure status of individuals, and in a community trial the unit of study is the group or population and the investigator intervenes to change the exposure status of whole groups or populations of people.

Clinical trials

In a *clinical trial* one group of individuals receive an intervention and are compared to another group who do not receive the intervention. Clinical trials are often divided into two types: therapeutic or secondary prevention trials, and preventive or primary prevention trials. Therapeutic trials are conducted among patients with a particular disease or health problem to determine the ability of an intervention (such as a drug, changes in diet, or psychological counselling) to reduce symptoms, prevent recurrence, or decrease the risk of death from that disease. A preventive trial is used to evaluate whether an intervention reduces the risk of developing a disease among those who are free from it when they enter the trial.

As in all epidemiological studies, bias is a potential problem, and one which must be guarded against in clinical trials. The gold standard design for clinical trials, i.e., that which is least prone to bias, is the *randomized* double blind controlled trial.

'*Randomized*' refers to the fact that subjects are assigned to the intervention or control group at random and that neither the investigator or subject has any say in who goes into which group. This avoids the potential bias of the investigator choosing subjects s/he feels would be most likely to benefit from the intervention for the intervention group, and a similar possible bias if the choice were left up to the subjects. Clearly for this to work, subjects must agree to take part in the study before randomization – if their agreement to participate is dependent upon which group they are randomized to this could also produce quite different types of subjects in the intervention and control groups. It is sometimes argued that surely it would be better for the investigator to decide who goes into the intervention and control groups because he or she could then make sure that the two groups are comparable rather than leaving it to chance. There are at least two reasons why randomization is still preferable. First, there may be unknown factors which could influence the outcome. Randomization ensures, within the limits of chance, that any such factors are evenly distributed between the intervention and control groups. Second, however hard the investigators try to produce two similar groups, it remains possible that they will be biased in their allocation of subjects, perhaps in ways of which they are not really aware. What may be done sometimes is to stratify the randomization process. For example, in a study with men and women it may be desirable to have the sexes equally distributed across the intervention and control groups. This could be achieved by undertaking the randomization in pairs of the same sex – one of the pair is assigned randomly to the intervention group and the other to the control group.

'*Double blind*' refers to the fact that neither the investigator nor the subject knows whether they are in the intervention group. Clearly this is not always possible for practical reasons. It is most obviously possible when the intervention is a drug. In this situation the intervention group can receive a tablet which contains the drug and the control group receive an identical looking, and ideally tasting, tablet which does not. With the correct organizational arrangements, neither the subjects nor the investigators need know who is receiving the intervention and who is not. Only at the end of the study would the 'code' be broken and the results analysed according to who had been taking the drug and who had not. The reason for going to all this trouble is to avoid the bias that may be introduced by the subjects' or the investigators' expectations about whether or not the drug works. Thus, for example, subjects who knew they were taking the tablet without the drug would not expect any benefit, where as subjects taking the tablet with the drug would. Because of this expectation, subjects taking the tablet with the drug may feel and report benefits even if the drug is of no use at all. This effect is known as the placebo effect. It is even possible to undertake what is sometimes called a triple blind study. This is the same as double blind but in addition the person undertaking the analysis doesn't know which is the control or intervention group.

Community trials

In a community trial the units of study are communities rather than individuals. This is particularly appropriate for diseases that have their origins in social, cultural or environmental conditions, where it makes sense to try and change these conditions on a community-wide basis rather than an individual basis. For example, a community trial aimed at changing diet might include widespread information campaigns using the local media, as well as measures to increase the availability of healthy foods in the local shops. There are two main limitations to community trials. The first is that it is usually only possible for practical reasons to include a small number of communities, making random allocation less likely to be successful in achieving comparable groups. Thus usually non-random allocation is used to try and ensure that the groups are comparable, matching the communities as far as possible on what are thought to be characteristics that may affect the outcome. The second limitation is that is almost impossible to isolate the control from the intervention communities. The control communities are almost bound to be aware of what is going on in the intervention community and may therefore also change.

Summary

Use the following questions to write your own summary:

1   Distinguish between what is meant by the terms descriptive, analytical and intervention when referring to types of epidemiological study.

2   Outline the design of studies you would use to do the following:
- evaluate whether a new drug is effective in treating a condition;

- examine the cause of death by age, sex and area of residence for people living in England last year;

- measure the amount of diabetes in a population;

- examine whether people exposed to an unusual industrial chemical are at an increased risk of developing certain diseases;

- determine whether a mass media campaign to encourage people to change an aspect of their life style is effective;

- identify possible causes of a rare disease.

Now reflect again on what your skills and knowledge currently are, where there are gaps and any actions arising.

Public health standards	
Surveillance & assessment	
Promoting & protecting	
Developing quality & risk management	
Collaborative working for health	
Developing programmes & services & reducing inequalities	
Policy & strategy development & implementation	
Working with & for communities	
Strategic leadership	
Research & Development	
Ethically managing self, people & resources	

6

Weighing up the evidence from epidemiological studies

Why are bias, confounding and chance possible explanations for an association found in an epidemiological study?

How can bias be minimized?

How can confounding be addressed?

What is meant by 'statistical significance'?

How can you assess the causality of an association?

After working through this chapter, you should be able to:

- discuss the roles of bias, confounding and chance as possible explanations for associations found in a study;
- outline how bias, confounding and chance can be addressed in the design or analysis of a study;
- compare and contrast the concepts of association and causality.

Association and causation

One of the main of uses of epidemiological studies is to identify associations between exposures and health outcomes. We commonly do this by computing relative risk, which is the incidence of the health outcome in those exposed divided by the incidence of the health outcome in those not exposed. For example, the incidence of lung cancer in heavy cigarette smokers is around 20 times higher than in non-smokers. This relative risk of 20 indicates a very strong association between cigarette smoking and lung cancer. You may be tempted to conclude from this fact alone that cigarette smoking causes lung cancer. However, this conclusion cannot be reached so easily. You must answer an important question first: Are you convinced that the association found between an exposure and an outcome in a study is real? There are many reasons why an association may be found in a particular study, when in fact no such association exists in the wider population. So in such a case the association was not real, it was an artefact. Such artefact may, for example, have been created by the way the study population was chosen from the wider population or by how exposures and outcomes were measured unequally. If you are convinced that it seems likely that the association you found is real, remember the aphorism, 'association does not mean causation'. When you assess whether an association is likely to be causal, you pass judgement on your findings in the light of all the evidence available to you from your own investigation and from investigations from others before you. You also include evidence published from disciplines other than epidemiology. This chapter introduces you to the process of deciding whether an association is real and then whether it is likely to be causal. However, before proceeding we must give some consideration to what is meant when we call something the 'cause' of a disease or other health state. We return to the example of Exercise 1.4 in Chapter 1 on the causes of tuberculosis.

The study of causality runs deep and remains the subject of much philosophical debate. A pragmatic approach to causality, which fits the aims of public health, is to refer to 'causes' of a disease as those factors which if modified, whether singly or in combination, lead to a change in the incidence of the disease. Now work through Exercise 6.1.

Exercise 6.1

What causes tuberculosis? Consider whether the following statements are true or false and give the reasons for your opinion:

1 Tuberculosis is caused by tuberculosis bacteria.

2 Tuberculosis is caused by poor housing, overcrowding, malnutrition and poverty.

3 Tuberculosis is caused by increased susceptibility to infection.

Without tuberculosis bacteria, tuberculosis (TB) cannot occur. They must be present. They are a *necessary cause* for anyone to contract tuberculosis. However, the exposure to tuberculosis bacteria alone is not a *sufficient cause*. For example, someone who is generally healthy and well nourished is not very likely to develop clinical tuberculosis after coming into contact with tuberculosis bacteria. Of course, much will also depend on the level and length of exposure, so if a person lives in over-crowded housing, they will be more likely to develop tuberculosis. Most causes that are of interest in the field of public health are not on their own sufficient to cause disease. They are components of sufficient causes. In the case of tuberculosis we know of several *component causes* that contribute to a person developing the disease. Environmental factors, such as overcrowding and malnutrition, are important. The susceptibility of the individual is important: an individual whose immune system is weakened by another disease is more susceptible to contract tuberculosis. Thus, poor living conditions, immunosuppression and tuberculosis bacteria are all component causes of TB, and together they may form *sufficient cause* (i.e., cause the disease). A number of conceptual models have been used to conceptualize this interplay of factors operating at various levels. Web of causation, interacting component cause model, wheel of causation and host–agent–environment are possibly the most important models.

To plan preventive action for health, it is not necessary to always identify all the components of a sufficient cause, because intervening in one component may be enough to break the chain of events. The metaphor of a black box has often been used to illustrate this. K. Rothman, the emminent American epidemiologist, uses the way a child learns to use a light switch to lighten up a room as an illustration in his introductory epidemiology teaching. The child may conclude that the flick of the switch causes the light to go on. But those who have learned their physics at school know that functioning light bulbs, the provision of electricity to the house, and wiring, are all required to make the switch turn the light on.

In the case of tuberculosis we know that death rates from the disease in England and Wales fell from almost 4000 per million people in 1840, to around 600 per million people in 1940, before any effective chemotherapy or vaccination was available. This decline seems to have been largely due to improvements in nutrition and housing conditions. Around 1840 many people were affected by malnutrition and were living in overcrowded and damp houses. With the decline in the prevalence of these component causes the incidence of TB declined because fewer people were exposed to sufficient cause. This example also illustrates that the strength of a causal risk factor is often dependent on the prevalence of other factors. For example, the risk of developing TB after exposure to the bacteria is higher in malnourished populations than in those that are well nourished.

Answering the question 'is the association real?'

Epidemiological research is not a laboratory science, it is conducted with humans living within their environment. This is both a strength and a weakness of epidemiology. It is a strength that people are observed within their natural environment. The weakness is that the epidemiological researcher has limited control over many of the factors influencing the health of individuals. This means that the epidemiologist has to assess whether an observed association is real or whether there are alternative explanations for it. Of course the converse is also the case – no association may be found even when in fact one exists. To help illustrate the process of making this assessment we will refer to a well-known study which examined the relationship between exposure to asbestos and deaths from lung cancer. In this study the causes of death diagnosed at autopsy of men employed in an asbestos works over a 20-year period (1933–52) were reviewed. The researcher calculated how many deaths would have been expected in total and from different causes if the workers had the same death rates of men in England and Wales over the same period of time. Some of the results from this study are shown in Table 6.1. While working through this example you will follow a framework which can be used to assess the nature of associations reported in any epidemiological study. This framework is illustrated in Figure 6.1. Look at this now before reading further.

Table 6.1 Causes of death among male asbestos workers compared with mortality experience of all men in England and Wales

Cause of death	Number of observed deaths	Number of deaths expected on England and Wales rates
Lung cancer	11	0.8
Neoplasm (other than lung cancer)	4	2.3
All causes	39	15.4

Source: Adapted from Doll, R. (1955) Mortality from lung cancer in asbestos workers, *British Medical Journal*, 12: 81–6.

Assessing the role of bias

Bias can be defined as any systematic error in an epidemiological study that results in an incorrect estimate of the association between an exposure and the occurrence of a disease. Last and Spasoff's (2000) *Dictionary of Epidemiology* calls it a deviation from the truth. Bias can be divided into two broad types: selection bias and information bias.

- Selection bias refers to any systematic error that arises when identifying or recruiting the subjects to the study. This can occur in several ways. For example, the people who volunteer to take part in a study may be quite different in a range of characteristics to those who do not. Thus those who agree to take part may not be representative of the population from which the sample was taken. This example of selection bias is called response bias.

- Information bias refers to systematic error which results from the way in which the data are collected. For example, in case-control studies (these are described in Chapter 5) data on exposure are usually collected retrospectively, often by interview. It is possible that people with the disease (cases) will report their history of exposure differently to those without, simply because the presence of the disease focuses the mind. This example of information bias is called recall bias, and may result in an association being found between an exposure and a disease when in fact none exists.

Another important source of error or bias arises if subjects erroneously are assigned to the wrong exposure group. In the example of lung cancer mortality

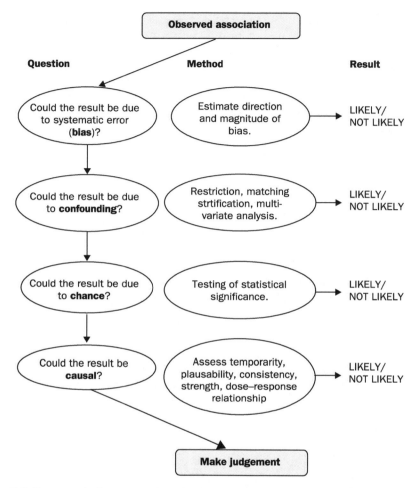

Figure 6.1 Framework for assessing the relationship between an association and an outcome

among asbestos workers this could be someone who did not remember that they worked with asbestos even though they had.

Bias creates wrong estimates of the associations between exposures and health outcomes. It can lead to either an over-estimation of risk or the failure to detect an association even if the truth is that one exists.

Look now at Exercise 6.2. This addresses some of the biases that were considered as possible explanations for the association between working with asbestos and death from lung cancer shown in Table 6.1.

Clearly the examples of potential bias given in Exercise 6.2 could all account for an apparent association between asbestos workers and lung cancer when none exists. Such potential biases were carefully considered by the author of the paper who

---

Exercise 6.2

Look at the results again in Table 6.1. Consider the following suggested biases and write down your view on whether or not they could be responsible for the association between working with asbestos and lung cancer:

• Asbestos workers were more likely to be incorrectly diagnosed as suffering from lung cancer than men in England and Wales.

• Lung cancer was insufficiently diagnosed in the general population compared to asbestos workers.

• Pathologists were more likely to report lung cancer in autopsies on asbestos workers compared to autopsies in the general population.

---

concluded that there was no evidence that such biases could account for the observed association.

Bias cannot be controlled for at the analysis stage of a study, it needs to be prevented and controlled through careful design of the study. The choice and recruitment of the study population, the methods of data collection, the sources of information about exposure and disease need to be carefully planned and executed to avoid bias.

Assessing the role of confounding

A second alternative explanation for an observed association is the mixing of effects by a third factor, which is associated with both the exposure and independently with the risk of developing the disease. This is called confounding. Work through Exercise 6.3 before reading further.

Exercise 6.3

Assume that all workers in the asbestos and lung cancer study were heavy smokers. Write down how you think this might have affected the results of the study.

If the proportion of smokers among the asbestos workers was much higher than the proportion of smokers in the general population, this could have accounted at least in part for the higher lung cancer rates among the workers. The researchers would have compared cases and controls that were not like with like. In 1955 when this study was published, smoking was not yet considered to be associated with lung cancer. Later studies in asbestos workers established that asbestos was associated with lung cancer independently from smoking, and found that smokers who worked with asbestos had an even higher risk of developing lung cancer than smokers who did not.

There are several methods to control for confounding in epidemiological studies. Some are applied when designing a study, others are used during the analysis of data. In an intervention study (described in the Chapter 5) subjects can be randomized to the intervention and control groups, so that is it will be equally likely that they get assigned into the intervention or the control group. Randomization will ensure, within the limits of chance, that confounding factors are evenly distributed between the intervention and control groups. There are, however, many situations where randomization cannot be applied, for example, because it would be unethical to offer treatment to some but not others. An alternative approach in the design of a study to control for confounding is to restrict your study sample to only those individuals who do not have a suspected or known confounding factor (restriction). For example, all smokers could have been excluded from the study of asbestos exposure and lung cancer. Disadvantages of restricting the sample include that the number whom you can be study might be too small to give a meaningful result, and that those studied may be quite atypical of the general exposed population. Often a better approach is to include all groups in the study, such as smokers and non-smokers, and then to look at those groups separately in the analysis, a method which is called stratification.

Another method of dealing with confounding is to look at subjects in matched pairs. In our asbestos–lung-cancer example we could form pairs between smokers who worked in the asbestos industry and smokers who did not work in the asbestos industry, and similarly with non-smokers. We could match for other variables as well. For example, we might match pairs on the basis of age, sex, social class as well as smoking status. The disadvantage of this approach is that it can be very difficult, time-consuming and therefore expensive. It can also present problems in finding enough people who can be matched.

Nowadays, with the power provided by personal computers, the most common approach to control for confounding is to use statistical methods during the analysis stage of a study. There are statistical techniques such as multivariate analysis which allow for the estimation of an association between an exposure and a disease while controlling for several confounding factors simultaneously.

Assessing the role of chance

The third alternative explanation for an observed association is that it has arisen by chance alone. Assessing the role of chance involves the use of a statistical approach known as hypothesis or significance testing. Space does not permit full justice to be done here to the process of significance testing and the assumptions on which it is based. Here the main steps in the process and the reasoning behind it are outlined. Table 6.2 contains the results shown in Table 6.1 but also contains an additional column showing the *p* value statistics for the difference between the observed and expected values. How these were derived and how they are interpreted are summarized below.

Table 6.2 Causes of death among male asbestos workers compared with mortality experience of all men in England and Wales, plus *p* values for the difference between the observed and expected deaths

Cause of death	Number of observed deaths	Number of deaths expected on England and Wales rates	Probability (p)
Lung cancer	11	0.8	$p < 0.001$
Neoplasm (other than lung cancer)	4	2.3	$p > 0.1$
All causes	39	15.4	$p < 0.001$

Source: Adapted from Doll, R. (1955) Mortality from lung cancer in asbestos workers, *British Medical Journal*, 12: 81–6.

Steps in testing statistical significance:

1 *State the research hypothesis.* In the case of asbestos exposure and lung cancer the research hypothesis might be framed as 'asbestos exposure is associated with lung cancer'.

2 *Formulate the statistical hypothesis.* The statistical hypothesis translates the research hypothesis into a form to which statistical tests can be applied. This is done by formulating what is called the null hypothesis. The null hypothesis states that the results observed in a study are no different from what might have occurred by chance alone. In the example of the study into asbestos exposure and lung cancer, the null hypothesis would be that there is no difference in the death rate from lung cancer in asbestos workers than in the general population. The test of statistical significance gives the probability of the observed results arising by chance. For example a significance level with a *p* value of 0.1 indicates that assuming the null hypothesis is correct, the probability of obtaining the result in the study, or a more extreme result, is 0.1 or 10 per cent. Put another way, simply by chance alone this result (or more extreme) would be expected in 10 per cent of cases.

3 *Specify the rules to evaluate the null hypothesis* It is common practice to specify a level of statistical significance against which to evaluate the null hypothesis. The most commonly used level of statistical significance is 5 per cent, also expressed as *p* less than 0.05. Thus if the level is below 5 per cent it is standard practice to reject the null hypothesis and to assume that the observed results are unlikely to be due to chance, and, conversely, if the level is above 5 per cent to accept the null hypothesis and assume that the results may well be due to chance. The lower the value of the *p*, the more we will be inclined to reject the null hypothesis.

4   *Carry out the analysis and interpret the statistics* The final steps of the testing for statistical significance are to compute the tests and to interpret the results. If you look at the *p* values in Table 6.2 you will see, for example, that the *p* value for lung cancer was less than 0.001, or 1 in 1000. This means that if the null hypothesis were true, the results obtained would be expected by chance alone on less than 1 in 1000 occasions. Thus the explanation that the association between lung cancer and asbestos workers was due to chance (the null hypothesis) was rejected.

It cannot be emphasized too strongly that the cut-off point of 5 per cent for statistical significance, or any other cut-off point that may be used, is entirely arbitrary, and that the inflexible use of an arbitrary cut-off point often makes a nonsense of the interpretation of data. It is common in medical papers to see significance levels as different as 0.051 and 0.8 both simply described as 'non-significant'. However, clearly the probability of obtaining a result by chance alone of 5.1 per cent conveys a very different picture to a probability of 80 per cent. Another problem inherent in the interpretation of a *p* value results from the fact that it reflects both the magnitude of any difference between the groups being compared and the size of the sample. A small difference in a large sample, and large difference in a small sample, can lead to similar *p* values. Today, many epidemiologists prefer to base statistical inference on what are called 'confidence intervals'. The confidence interval reports a range of values which have a specified probability of containing the true value. In Table 6.2 confidence intervals could be put on the size of the difference between the observed and the expected number of deaths. This would convey information on the likelihood of observing that difference by chance but in addition it would also convey information on where the true difference may lie.

Finally, you need to appreciate that statistical significance is by no means equivalent to clinical importance. A small effect may be statistically significant if the size of the sample studied is large, but be of little clinical importance. Conversely a large effect may fail to reach statistical significance if the sample size is small, but potentially be of great importance for health.

When does association mean causation?

Once you have established an association between an exposure and a disease (or other health outcome), and you have carefully considered and ruled out bias, confounding and chance as likely explanations, the next step is to make a judgement as to whether the association is likely to be causal. There is no watertight method of making such a judgement. A number of criteria have been suggested which, taken together, can strengthen or weaken the case that the association is causal. These include:

- *The strength of the association* – a strong association (e.g., with a large relative risk) is less likely to be due to undetected biases than a weak association. But a weak association could still be causal.
- *Consistency* – finding the same association in different studies, on different

populations under different circumstances. But some causes may only operate in specific circumstances.

- *Temporality* – the cause must precede the effect in time. No 'buts' for this criterion.

- *Dose-response relationship* – This means to say that a causal relationship is likely to show a dose-response relationship: the greater the exposure, the greater the chance of the disease. This certainly holds true for cigarette smoking and lung cancer. But for some causes any (even a very small exposure) exposure may be enough to cause disease, and conversely a dose – response relationship could still be due to confounding.

- *Biological plausibility* – This refers to any evidence of known biological mechanisms by which the exposure could cause the disease? But clearly lack of an obvious mechanism does not mean it cannot be causal, because the mechanism may still need to be discovered

- *Experimental evidence* – may be available from experiments on animals but unlikely to present for humans. But what appears causal in a laboratory rat may be of little relevance to humans.

The short answer to the question 'when does association mean causation?' is that it is hard to say. It is a judgement. The above criteria can help in the process of judgement but apart from temporality (to be causal an exposure must precede the disease), none of them present hard and fast rules. This may seem an unsatisfactory situation but it is not an excuse for inaction. This was summed up nicely by Austin Bradford Hill, the British statistician who first suggested the criteria listed above. He wrote: 'All scientific work is incomplete [and] is liable to be upset or modified by advancing knowledge. That does not confer upon us a freedom to ignore the knowledge we already have, or to postpone the action that it appears to demand at a given time.'

Summary

Write your own summary using the following questions and headings:

1   What is meant by the terms bias and confounding and why are they possible explanations for an association found in an epidemiological study?

2   Describe ways in which bias and confounding can be addressed.

3   What is meant by the term 'null hypothesis' and how is it used to assess the role of chance in explaining an association found in an epidemiological study?

4   How would you assess the causality of an association?

Now reflect again on what your skills and knowledge currently are, where there are gaps and any actions arising.

Public health standards	
Surveillance & assessment	
Promoting & protecting	
Developing quality & risk management	
Collaborative working for health	
Developing programmes & services & reducing inequalities	
Policy & strategy development & implementation	
Working with & for communities	
Strategic leadership	
Research & Development	
Ethically managing self, people & resources	

7

The determinants of health and disease

What are proximal and distal determinants of disease?

How does the health of populations in the poorest parts of the world differ from those in the richest?

After working through this chapter, you should be able to:

- discuss what is meant by determinants and causes of disease;
- provide definitions of proximal and distal determinants, and necessary and sufficient causes;
- discuss the nature of the relationship between poverty and poor health;
- provide a critical account of the theory of the epidemiological transition;
- give an overview of the demographic characteristics and disease patterns in different parts of the world.

Start this chapter by reading through Exercise 7.1.

Proximal and distal determinants of health and disease

In epidemiology and public health the word 'determinant' is used to refer to any factor, whether an event, characteristic, or other definable entity, that brings about, or contributes to, a change in health. It is common to refer to proximal and distal determinants. A distal determinant is one that is remote, either in position, time or resemblance to the outcome of concern, and a proximal determinant is one that is much closer to the outcome of concern. For example, in the case of Jason's cut and infected leg, the proximal determinants include the fact that he fell on some dirty, sharp, jagged steel. The more distal determinants include the fact that there was nowhere else to play in that neighbourhood, and he lives in that neighbourhood

---

Exercise 7.1

'Why is Jason in the hospital?'

> Because he has a bad infection in his leg.
> But why does he have an infection?
> Because he has a cut on his leg and it got infected.
> But why does he have a cut on his leg?
> Because he was playing in the junk yard next to his apartment building and there
>   was some sharp, jagged steel there that he fell on.
> But why was he playing in a junk yard?
> Because his neighbourhood is kind of run down. A lot of kids play there and there is
>   no one to supervise them.
> But why does he live in that neighbourhood?
> Because his parents can't afford a nicer place to live.
> But why can't his parents afford a nicer place to live?
> Because his Dad is unemployed and his Mom is sick.
> But why is his Dad unemployed?
> Because he doesn't have much education and he can't find a job.
> But why . . .?
>   (Public Health Agency of Canada website: www.phac-aspc.gc.ca/)

What actions would you advocate to reduce the rate of childhood accidents in this neighbourhood?

---

because his parents are too poor to live elsewhere. Figure 7.1 illustrates the different levels and types of determinants of health and disease, with the more distal determinants on the outside, working in towards more proximal determinants.

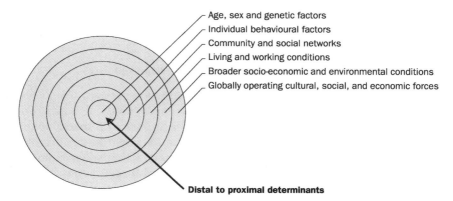

Age, sex and genetic factors
Individual behavioural factors
Community and social networks
Living and working conditions
Broader socio-economic and environmental conditions
Globally operating cultural, social, and economic forces

Distal to proximal determinants

Figure 7.1 Different levels and types of determinants of health and disease (based on a figure from the Public Health Agency of Canada)

One of the strongest and most pervasive distal determinants of health is socio-economic circumstances. It is estimated that around one-sixth of the world's 6.2 billion population live in extreme poverty, on less than the equivalent of $1 a day, and for them it is a daily struggle to meet the basic necessities of life. It is hardly surprising therefore that overall people in this situation have the worst health experience in the world.

What perhaps is more surprising is that even in the world's richest countries, such as those of North America and Western Europe, people who are less well off have substantially shorter life expectancies and more illnesses that the richer members of those countries. In fact the differences by socio-economic circumstances are finely graded, there is no threshold: life expectancy increases, and rates of illness decline across the spectrum from the poorest to the richest members of society. Work through Exercise 7.2, which shows the differences in life expectancy at birth across occupational class groups in England and Wales.

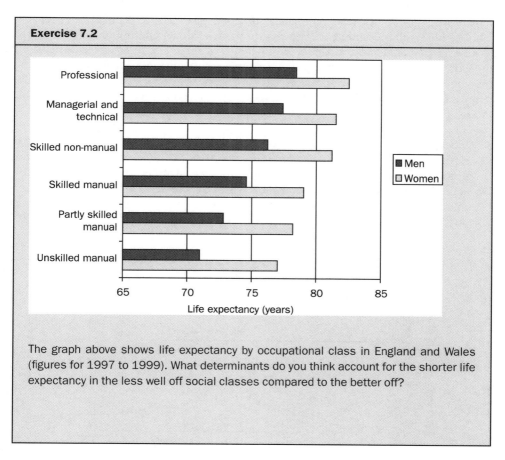

Exercise 7.2

The graph above shows life expectancy by occupational class in England and Wales (figures for 1997 to 1999). What determinants do you think account for the shorter life expectancy in the less well off social classes compared to the better off?

It is likely that a number of factors related to socio-economic circumstances contribute to these differences in life expectancy by occupational and social class shown in Exercise 7.2. They include: absolute and relative material deprivation, differences in education and behaviours related to health, such as smoking and aspects of diet and long-term psychological stress. These factors do not operate at one point in time, and it is increasingly clear that the risk of many adverse health outcomes is related to exposures that have occurred throughout life, even during growth in the womb.

Determinants over the life course

The recognition that exposure to disadvantageous experiences and environments in earlier life increase the risk of poorer health in later life, has led to the development of a new approach to the study of the risk of disease in adults, one that is called 'life course epidemiology'. Life course epidemiology can be defined as the study of the long-term effects on disease risk of physical and social exposures during gestation, childhood, adolescence, young adulthood and later life.

The simplest way to think of disease determinants operating over the life course is the accumulation of adverse experiences that increase the risk of disease in later life. This is illustrated in Figure 7.2. The risk of disease will depend not only on exposure to adverse personal and broader economic/environmental circumstances but also on the genetic make-up of the individual. In some individuals the accumulation of risk may never be enough to cause a particular disease. However, for most health outcomes the situation is likely to be more complex than this simple risk accumulation model. For example:

- There is evidence that there are critical periods of development during which adverse exposures have a greater influence than at other times. Thus, low for gestational age birth weight, thought to be due to poor nutrition in-utero, is related to the risk of diabetes and cardiovascular disease as an adult. It is thought that influences during foetal development have a programming effect on glucose and lipid metabolism and blood pressure levels.

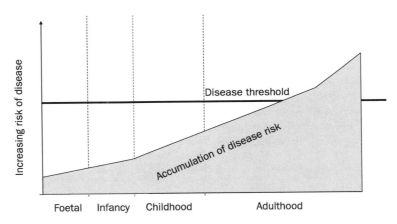

Figure 7.2 Simple model illustrating accumulation of disease risk over the life course, with disease occurring once a threshold is crossed

- Exposures at different stages of the life course may interact with each other. For example, there is evidence that it is the combination of low birth weight followed by overweight and obesity in childhood that particularly increases the risk of cardiovascular disease in later life.

- Adverse exposures at one stage of life need not be carried over to a later stage, at least not fully. For example, for middle-aged adults who stop smoking, the risk of adverse health consequences associated with smoking falls within a few years to close to those of lifelong non-smokers.

Determinants or causes?

There is clearly a great deal of overlap between what is meant by 'a determinant' of a health state and what is meant by 'a cause' of a health state. Indeed, the words are often used interchangeably and you may see one used to help define the other. However, in epidemiology, and in the approach taken in this book, the word 'cause' tends to be reserved for those factors that have been rigorously evaluated, along the lines described at the end of Chapter 5, and for which there is strong and consistent evidence that they lead to a specific health outcome. Factors that have been subjected to the type of rigorous evaluation described in Chapter 5 are more likely to be in the class of proximal determinants, not least because these are easier to evaluate in this way.

It can be useful to consider causes as 'necessary' and 'sufficient'. A 'necessary cause' is one which must be present for the health outcome to occur. A good example is a specific infectious agent, such as the tuberculosis bacillus. This must be present for the disease tuberculosis to occur. However, exposure to the bacillus alone is not sufficient to cause the disease. Other factors determine whether the disease will occur. These include the nature and length of exposure to the bacillus and the immune status of the individual, which in turn may be related to other factors such as long-term heavy alcohol consumption, the presence of diabetes or infection with HIV. The term 'sufficient cause' is used to refer to a factor, or more usually a combination of factors, that inevitably produce a particular health outcome. Although the concepts of 'necessary' and 'sufficient' causes are useful, our knowledge of these causes, as strictly defined, for many diseases and other health states is very limited.

We hope that the preceding sections on disease determinants have helped to illustrate the multilayered and interrelated nature of the determinants of health states. Even where a necessary cause is known, as for an infectious disease, the reasons why a particular individual or group of individuals are affected by that disease, and others are not, is dependent on a range of determinants.

Patterns of diseases over time and in the world today

The theory of the epidemiological transition

There have been huge increases in life expectancy in many countries over the past 100 to 200 years, but there continue to be huge differences in health between different populations around the world, with the worst health in its poorest parts. The theory of the epidemiological transition, described below, provides a framework for considering the role of, and the interaction between, distal and proximal determinants in driving changes in health over time.

The theory of the epidemiological transition was developed in order to provide an overall framework for considering changes in population fertility and mortality (demographic change), the relationship of these to disease patterns, and the relationship of both of these to economic, social and technological changes. It was developed through a study of the experience of several countries. The relationships between these various factors are summarized in Figure 7.3. A variety of factors form the basis of this process. They include rising incomes, industrialization and urbanization, improved access to education, particularly for women, and public and personal health measures. The relative importance of these has differed over time and between populations. For example, as was illustrated in Chapter 1, many of the improvements in public health in nineteenth- and early twentieth-century England had little to do with medical knowledge and services, and more to do with improvements in economic circumstances, improved sanitation and living conditions (such as nutrition, housing and personal hygiene). However, today there are some highly effective medical interventions that can have a large impact on population health. They include childhood immunization, oral rehydration therapy for vomiting and diarrhoea, and skilled antenatal care.

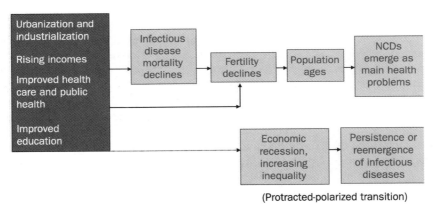

(Protracted-polarized transition)

Figure 7.3 Representation of the epidemiological transition

Note: NCDs – chronic, noncommunicable diseases.

The demographic changes described in the epidemiological transition are the result of falling mortality, particularly in infants and young children, and falling fertility. Together these lead to a greater proportion of the population being made up of people in older age groups. Over time the population age structure moves from the 'pyramid' still seen in low income countries today to the 'stack' seen in most rich countries (see, for example, Figure 3.2 in Chapter 3). As the population becomes older, they develop the chronic diseases associated with aging, such as cardiovascular disease and cancers. Omran, who first proposed the theory of the epidemiological transition, identified three broad mortality patterns as populations move through the transition.

He called these respectively:

- 'the age of pestilence and famine', with a high fluctuating mortality that prevents sustained population growth;
- 'the age of receding pandemics', when mortality declines progressively and the rate of decline accelerates as epidemic peaks disappear;
- 'the age of degenerative and man-made diseases', with a continuing mortality decline towards stability at a relatively low level, and with this phase representing the time at which non-communicable diseases become the main health problems within a population.

In 1986, Olshansky and Ault proposed a fourth stage:

- 'the age of delayed degenerative diseases', to describe the change from chronic noncommunicable diseases afflicting adults between their 30s and 50s to pre-dominantly afflicting elderly adults, between their 60s and 80s. This is now the case for most populations living in Western European, North American and some other countries such as Japan, Australia and New Zealand.

In addition to these different stages of the transition process, four main models, or versions, of the overall process have been described: classical, delayed, polarized and accelerated. These models describe different rates of moving through the stages described above, ranging from one or more centuries in the classical model to a few decades in the accelerated model. The models also reflect that some populations continue to have high levels of infectious disease even as NCDs emerge (the delayed model) and that in some populations (usually those with marked economic inequal-ity), subgroups are at different stages (the polarized model). Both the delayed and polarized models are particularly apt for many of world's poorest countries today.

The two-way relationship between economic and social development and health

The diagram of the epidemiological transition, Figure 7.3, is misleading in one very important way. It implies that the relationship between economic and social develop-ment is one way, when there is clearly a two-way relationship. In some of the poorest parts of the world, particularly in Africa, the extremely high burden of disease stands as a barrier to economic development. Measures aimed at reducing specific diseases, while justified of course on the grounds of relieving human suffering, are also an essential part of a programme to promote economic and social development. For example, at the time of writing, roughly one-sixth of the world's population lives in extreme poverty, on the equivalent of less than $1 per day. The life expectancy of people living in extreme poverty is around 30 years less than the sixth richest propor-tion of the world's population. Major contributors to this difference in life expectancy are the following: maternal and perinatal mortality, vaccine-preventable diseases, acute respiratory infections and diarrhoea, protein, energy and micronutrient malnutrition, malaria and HIV/AIDS. All of these conditions are either wholly or largely preventable or treatable. Implementing public health measures to reduce death and disability from these conditions is seen by the World Health Organization and United Nations as central to promoting social and economic development among the world's poor and reducing extreme poverty.

The influence of globalization

Today, more than ever, economic, social and technological changes all over the world are driven by forces of globalization. The term 'globalization' is used here to refer to the increasing interconnectedness of populations through the flow of services, money, goods, ideas and people across national borders.

Globalization can have both positive and negative consequences for health. On the positive side, giving poor countries *fair* access to international trade can have a major impact on economic growth and improved standards of living and health, as has been seen in recent years in large parts of India and China. Another example on the positive side is the exchange and dissemination of effective medical technologies. However, on the negative side the potential benefits of globalization are currently failing to reach millions of the world's poor, and some of the current terms and conditions of trade work against poor countries in favour of the rich. Increased movements of people provide new opportunities for the spread of disease, such as was evident in 2004 in the SARs (severe acute respiratory syndrome) outbreaks. In addition, the spread of some ideas and behaviours, almost always backed by powerful commercial interests, can be positively damaging to health, such as the promotion of smoking, alcohol consumption and high fat, high calorie, diets.

A note of caution on the theory of the epidemiological transition

The theory of the epidemiological transition is sometimes mistakenly seen as providing a set of laws to predict the future. It does not. It provides a useful framework for considering the interrelationships between demography, disease patterns and social and economic conditions. The nature and relative importance of these relationships are likely to differ between populations and over time. New and unforeseen factors complicate efforts to extrapolate from the experience of other populations who have gone through the epidemiological transition. The HIV pandemic, changes in political and economic systems, such as occurred with the dissolution of the Soviet Union, and the ravages of armed conflict, are but three examples of major unpredictable determinants of disease patterns.

Before going on to read about health and disease patterns in the world today, use your knowledge of the theory of the epidemiological transition, and your general knowledge, in Exercise 7.3 (facing).

Health and disease patterns in the world today

The contrast between the health experience of populations in the poorest parts of the world and those in the richest parts is stark and shocking. The matter-of-fact descriptions that follow cannot begin to touch the depth of suffering and grinding

---

Exercise 7.3

The next section of this chapter provides an overview of health and disease patterns in different parts of the world today. It does this by describing the situation for the poorest countries (low income), the richest (high income) and those in between (middle income). Using the theory of the epidemiological transition and knowledge of the relationship between poverty and disease rates, complete the following table indicating which group of countries has the highest, middle and lowest for each of the items.

Countries	% of population aged over 65 years	% of population living in cities	% of deaths due to non-communicable diseases	Life expectancy at birth	Average number of births per woman
Low income					
Middle income					
High income					

Now read on and see if all your answers are correct.

---

toil that is the lot of hundreds of millions of the world's poor, around one billion of whom survive on less than $1 a day. At the time of writing this chapter we were reminded through campaigns to coincide with the G8 summit of 2005 that every three seconds a child dies from a preventable disease. Equally, however, the descriptions that follow cannot capture the often remarkable resilience and determination of people living under such conditions to build a better life for themselves and their children.

In order to provide a broad global picture, descriptions are largely based on the World Bank classification of countries, based on their economies, into low income, middle income and high income. This classification is based on gross national income (GNI) per capita per year as estimated by the World Bank. The levels of GNI, based on figures for 2004, for the three categories are as follows:

- *Low income*: up to $825 per capita per year. Examples of countries in this category include the vast majority of countries in Sub-Saharan Africa, India, Pakistan, Bangladesh, parts of South-East Asia such as Vietnam and Cambodia and, in Europe, Moldova.
- *Middle income*: $826 to $10,065 per capita per year. Examples include most of the countries in Eastern Europe and Central Asia; Russia; most of the countries

in Central and South America; countries in parts of South-East Asia, including Thailand, Malaysia and Indonesia; many of the countries in the Middle East and most of the countries in the Caribbean.

- *High income*: $10,066 and above per capita per year. Examples include the countries of Western Europe, North America, Australia and New Zealand, Japan and several of the countries in the Middle East.

Obviously, each of these categories is broad, and you will sometimes see the low income category further divided into least developed countries and other low income, and the middle income into lower and upper-middle income.

Demographic characteristics

Less than one-sixth of the world's 6.2 billion people (figure for 2002) live in high income countries, with roughly half on the reminder living in low, and half in middle, income countries (see Table 7.1). Over one in three of the population in low income countries is aged less than 15 years of age, compared to less than one in five of the population in high income countries. Conversely over one in seven of people in high income countries are over 65 years of age compared to less than one in 20 in low income countries. The vast majority of people in high income countries live in urban areas, whereas the vast majority in low income countries live in rural areas.

Life expectancy at birth (the average length of life if current age and sex specific death rates apply) in low income countries is just under 60 years, almost 20 years less than in high income countries. In some of the poorest low income countries, such as those of Sub-Saharan Africa, life expectancy at birth is under 50 years, 30 years less than in high income countries. The total fertility rate (average number of births per woman) tends to be highest in the poorest countries and lowest in the richest. As described in the theory of the epidemiological transition, improvements in economic conditions and life expectancy tend to be associated with lower fertility rates. Thus fertility rates are highest in the least developed countries, the poorest of the low income countries, where the total fertility rate is 5.1 births per woman.

Table 7.1 Population data by income level

Income level	Population (millions)	% living in urban areas	% of population under 15	% of population aged 65 and above	Life expectancy at birth (years)	Total fertility rate (number of births per woman)
Low	2561	31.2	37.0	4.3	59.2	3.7
Middle	2721	52.8	26.3	7.0	70.1	2.1
High	941	77.8	18.3	14.6	78.4	1.7

Note: All figures from the *United Nations Human Development Indicators* as published in 2004 (see list in Further reading).

Risk of death and causes of death

The lower life expectancy in low income countries, compared to middle and high income countries, reflects higher death rates at all ages of life. The differences are particularly marked in infants and young children. Table 7.2 shows that the mortality in infants and children under 5 is over 15 times higher in low compared to high income countries, and five to six times higher in middle income countries. Infant and under-5 mortality in the least developed countries is 20 times higher than in high income countries. Although, the relative differences are less marked, the higher mortality continues throughout the rest of childhood and into adulthood. For example, Table 7.2 shows at the current death rates 45 per cent of men in low income countries will die before they are 65 (59 per cent of men in the least developed countries), compared to just under 20 per cent in high income countries.

Table 7.2 Infant, under-5 and mortality before the age of 65 years

Income	Infant mortality (per 1000 live births)	Under-5 years mortality (per 1000 live births)	Probability of dying before age 65 years (%)	
			Women	Men
Low	80	120	38.9	45.9
Middle	30	37	20.5	31.6
High	5	7	10.5	18.1

Note: All figures from the United Nations Human Development Indicators as published in 2004 (see list in Further reading).

The per centage of deaths by broad cause is shown in Figure 7.4. The broad categories, used by the World Health Organization and the World Bank in the Global Burden of Disease Study, are:

1   Communicable, maternal, perinatal and nutritional conditions: including all infectious diseases, deaths in women related to pregnancy, perinatal deaths, which include still births and deaths within the first week of life, and nutritional conditions such as protein-energy malnutrition and vitamin A deficiency.
2   Non-communicable diseases: covering cardiovascular diseases, cancers, endocrine conditions, such as diabetes, and neuropsychiatric disorders, which includes alcohol and drug use disorders.
3   Injuries, which include unintentional injuries, such as road traffic accidents, and intentional injuries, such as suicide and violence against others.

The major difference between the three groups of countries is that in the poorest countries of children and adults up to the age of 60, a much higher proportion of deaths are due to first category of conditions. Of the 18 million deaths worldwide due to these conditions in 2002, around 24 per cent were due to HIV infection or tuberculosis, and 22 per cent due to respiratory infections. Diarrhoeal diseases, mainly in infants and children, and vaccine-preventable diseases, such as whooping cough,

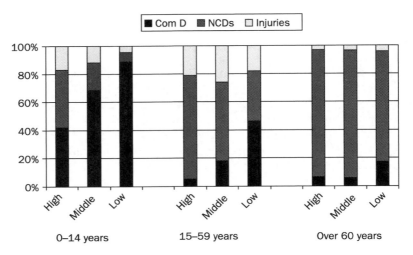

Figure 7.4 Percentages of deaths by broad cause and age for high, middle and low income countries

Note: See text for further details.

measles and tetanus, account for around 16 per cent of these deaths, and a further 13 per cent are related to low birth weight and problems at the time of birth. Seven per cent of deaths in this group are due to malaria.

The second group of conditions, noncommunicable diseases, accounted for 34 million deaths worldwide in 2002, 50 per cent of which were due to cardiovascular diseases, mainly ischaemic heart disease and cerebrovascular disease. Malignant neoplasms accounted for 21 per cent of deaths, respiratory diseases, such as chronic obstructive pulmonary disease and asthma, 11 per cent, and digestive diseases, such as peptic ulcer and cirrhosis of the liver, 6 per cent.

The last group of conditions, injuries, accounted for 5 million deaths in 2002. Of these deaths 69 per cent were classified as 'unintentional', including road traffic accidents (23 per cent of the 5 million) and falls (8 per cent). Thirty-one per cent were classified as 'intentional', including self-inflicted (17 per cent of the 5 million), violence (11 per cent) and war (3 per cent).

Taking into account mortality *and* morbidity

Focusing on causes of death as the main approach to describing the health status of populations gives little prominence to those conditions that have a low mortality but which cause substantial morbidity. In the Global Burden of Disease Study a single figure was derived for each disease that attempted to account for both its mortality and morbidity: the disability adjusted life year (DALY, for short). Very briefly, the number of DALYs for each condition is based on the number of years of potential life lost (compared to potential life expectancy), through mortality, or the number of years of healthy life lost, through living with the condition. This requires knowledge of, or an estimate of, the mortality from the condition and of the number of people living with it and how severely this affects their health. Inevitably this involves a large measure of judgement for many conditions. Details on the methods used by the Global Burden of Disease Study, and some criticism of the methods, can be found in some of the resources listed on pp. 164–5.

Using DALYs rather than deaths increases the relative importance of communicable and the other conditions in category one. Thus, globally these conditions accounted for 32 per cent of deaths in 2002 but for 41 per cent of DALYs. This is largely because several of the conditions in this category particularly affect infants and children and when not fatal can cause substantial long-term disability. Examples include perinatal conditions and malaria.

There are three categories of conditions in the noncommunicable disease group which have a low mortality but which are substantial causes of morbidity. Neuropsychiatric conditions are estimated to cause 2 per cent of all deaths but 13 per cent of all DALYs, with over a third of these DALYs being attributed to unipolar depression. Sense organ diseases, such as loss of vision and hearing are estimated to directly cause a tiny fraction of deaths, less than 0.01 per cent, but 5 per cent of all DALYs. Similarly musculoskeletal diseases cause less than 0.2 per cent of deaths but over 2 per cent of all DALYs.

Summary

Write your own summary of this chapter by working through the exercise and questions below:

1   Briefly summarize what is meant by each of the following:

   • proximal and distal determinants of disease;

   • necessary and sufficient causes of a disease.

2   What is meant by 'life course epidemiology'?

3   Briefly outline the theory of the epidemiological transition. How useful do you think it is in understanding demographic and disease patterns in the world today?

4   Use the box below to think through the proximal and distal determinants of three diseases or conditions, within a specific setting (i.e., place and population group), of which you have some knowledge. Try to pick contrasting conditions, such as affecting different age groups and being of particular importance in different population groups or parts of the world. Don't worry if you are unable to

list determinants under each of the six categories, complete as many as seem appropriate.

Disease or condition	1	2	3
Setting:			
Determinants Age, sex, genes:			
Individual behaviours:			
Community and social networks:			
Living and working conditions:			
Broader socio-economic and environmental factors:			
Globally operating factors:			

5   Give examples of conditions which cause a substantial burden of ill health but have a low mortality.

Now reflect again on what your skills and knowledge currently are, where there are gaps and any actions arising:

Public health standards	
Surveillance & assessment	
Promoting & protecting	
Developing quality & risk management	
Collaborative working for health	
Developing programmes & services & reducing inequalities	
Policy & strategy development & implementation	
Working with & for communities	
Strategic leadership	
Research & Development	
Ethically managing self, people & resources	

8

Health promotion

What do we mean by the term 'health promotion'?

Is health promotion the same as health education and health protection?

Are there different types of or approaches to health promotion?

Who should take responsibility for promoting health – the state or the individual?

How can we evaluate health promotion activities?

After working through this chapter you should be able to:

- distinguish the activities of health education, health protection, health promotion;
- identify the five models of health education;
- identify individual and collective responsibilities for health and debate where the balance should lie;
- identify trends in health promotion practice;
- identify factors to consider when evaluating health promotion;
- reflect on your own health promotion practice.

What do we mean by the term 'health promotion'?

The term 'health promotion' is used to describe a number of different activities. They all share a similar intent of promoting and improving health. There are different types of activity that are guided by different principles and that have different aims. We need to consider exactly what we mean by health promotion and what types of activities come under this heading.

Let's look at the two words in the phrase, 'health' and 'promotion'. It would be inappropriate to spend time trying to define health, suffice to say that the definition used sets the parameters for what is to be promoted. Work through Exercise 8.1 now.

Exercise 8.1

Give some thought to what you understand by the term health promotion by writing your own definition in the space below.

Your definition may have included:

- aspects of physical, psychological and social and mental health;
- prevention of disease processes;
- development of fitness;
- individual, group or society activities;
- education relating to health matters;
- achievement of individual or community health potential.

It would not be surprising if your definition gave considerable focus to healthy lifestyle issues, because this is a very common interpretation of health promotion. However, it is a mistake to think that spreading the word about healthy lifestyle options is all health promotion is about. Despite this, the healthy lifestyle discourse has been the dominant approach in practice and policy. However, more recently other dimensions such as social capacity and healthy communities are becoming more prominent. This widening approach still only addresses some health promotion options.

Dahlgren and Whitehead's (1991) model of the influences on health identified several layers or levels of influence that are presented in an adapted format here (see also the previous chapter on determinants of health, which includes a similar model of influences on health).

General socio-economic, Cultural, Environmental *actions*

Education, Food Production, Water & Sanitation, Health Care Services

Social & Community Factors

Individual Lifestyle Factors

Figure 8.1 Influences on health

Source: Adapted from Dahlgren and Whitehead (1991)

Criticism has been made that as you move away from the individual level, health becomes a weaker influence compared to other factors such as economics. Work through Exercise 8.2.

Exercise 8.2

Select one key lifestyle issue often emphasized in health promotion activity, e.g. smoking, diet, alcohol consumption, exercise levels.

Consider how this issue is addressed in your country at each of the levels highlighted in Dahlgren and Whitehead's (1991) model.

Is health the key factor influencing decision-making?

We'll return to these issues and discuss them in more detail later in the chapter.

Consider the World Health Organisation's (WHO) definition of health promotion:

> Health promotion is the process of enabling people to increase control over, and to improve, their health . . . Health is a positive concept emphasizing social and personal resources, as well as physical capacities. Therefore, health promotion is not just the responsibility of the health sector, but goes beyond healthy lifestyles to well-being.
>
> (Ottowa Charter 1986)

This statement widens the definition of health promotion considerably from the healthy lifestyle focus. It raises some important issues for consideration such as:

- What do we mean by enabling and how does it happen?
- If health promotion is not just the responsibility of the health sector – who else has responsibility?

Now do Exercise 8.3.

Exercise 8.3

Think about the concept of enabling – write down your understanding below. Reflect on your health promotion practice or that of others and consider if, and how, enabling is part of the process.

Depending on your individual role you may have identified that there are limitations to how much you can enable. It may be that the enabling process has to be facilitated at multiple levels. We can use the example of encouraging physical exercise to explore this a bit further:

- at one level people need to be enabled to appreciate the relevance of adequate levels of physical exercise for them as individuals;
- at another level the environment has to be cared for and safe to make an exercise such as walking inviting;
- transport systems and costs have to be such that opting not to use private transport is a viable option;
- facilities such as schools and shops need to be located within walking distance of housing estates;
- the cost of accessing leisure facilities needs to be affordable.

When you review this list, it is probably safe to say that no one person or sector can enable at every level.

What types of activities fall under the umbrella of health promotion?

Let's explore some of the components of health promotion further. We are all exposed to 'health promotion' in several different ways:

- on an individual basis;
- as part of a targeted group by, e.g., gender, age, lifestyle or location;
- initiated by the individual;
- imposed on the individual;
- in changes to the wider environment in which we live, e.g., banning smoking in public places;
- population-wide provision that is provided, e.g., health protection activities.

To consider the components of health promotion further, work through Exercise 8.4.

Exercise 8.4

Think about your own experiences and list how and when you consider you were exposed to health promotion. These experiences can go as far back or be as recent as you wish.

Your list probably includes aspects of health maintenance, health education, health enhancement, health protection and illness prevention. Health promotion is commonly used interchangeably with these other terms. Health promotion may include elements of all these activities, but not as an aim in themselves, but as a means of promoting optimum wellness.

Let's give some consideration to what we mean by some of the terms we've identified.

1   *Health education* can be thought of as giving information, instruction, or enhancing understanding about health. This could take the form of education about our health potential and about how to attain it or about how to avoid certain ill health problems.

Examples of this approach would include:

- encouraging individuals or communities to put health on their personal agenda;
- advising parents about childcare and development so that they can take appropriate child safety measures and so reduce the risk of accidents;
- encouraging adults to restrict their alcohol intake to avoid ill health consequences/road traffic accidents;
- encouraging individuals or communities to consider their health as opposed to ill health concerns and to put health onto their personal agenda;
- think of another example that is relevant to your interests and write down here:

_____

_____

You may have noticed that a significant amount of health education efforts focus on negative or ill health. In other words they don't often focus on enhancing health, but preventing or correcting health problems, i.e., encouraging participation in exercise to prevent coronary heart disease or even as part of a rehabilitation programme after coronary heart problems have been experienced. This is closely related to the next category – ill health prevention.

2   *Ill health prevention* can be thought of as increasing understanding of the factors contributing to the development of ill health so that preventative action may be taken to avoid or reduce exposure to them. Again, several types of activities could be involved:

- screening to identify disease at an early stage;
- developmental surveillance of the child population to identify deviations from normal at an early stage;
- increasing understanding of the causality of certain diseases and possible preventative actions, i.e., dental caries and diet, cigarette smoking and lung disease, social isolation and depression;
- immunization against certain diseases;
- again, identify some examples of your own:

_____

_____

Illness prevention activities are often categorized into at least three distinct levels. The definitions used here are based on epidemiological terms:

- primary prevention – action to prevent disease occurring, i.e., to reduce its incidence;
- secondary prevention – action to reduce the prevalence of a disease by shortening its duration, i.e., curing people who have the disease. Much screening activity, such as screening for breast cancer, is secondary prevention in that it aims to pick up the disease in its early stages to stand a better chance of effecting a cure;
- tertiary prevention – aims to reduce the complications (including disability and handicap) of a disease. Rehabilitation of individuals after a stroke is an example of tertiary prevention.

3 *Health legislation* relates to legislation to protect health by attempts to take the decision of participating in the activity out of the control of the individual. An example of such an activity would be legislation for seatbelt use, materials permitted for use in toy productions, tread levels on car tyres.

4 *Health protection* was the term previously used to describe a sub-set of health promotion and largely referred to legislative type activities. Recently its meaning has changed and the term health protection is now used in relation to three key activities:

- Protecting the population from infectious diseases. This includes the surveillance of infectious disease occurrence by making them notifiable. It also includes the tracing of contacts of patients with an infectious disease in order to provide advice or administer medication that prevents them from becoming ill and from spreading the disease to others.
- Protecting the population from harm resulting from chemical, poisons or radiation hazards. This includes the requirement for regular testing of drinking water and investigation of alleged clusters of disease that people attribute to environmental causes.
- Preparing for new and emerging threats such as bio-terrorism

5 *Health maintenance actions* can be thought of as those activities that help to perpetuate and sustain health-promoting activities. Examples could include:

- supporting and encouraging a mother to continue to breast feed her baby.
- reinforcing good dietary habits.
- again, identify some examples of your own:
- _____
- _____

Models of health education and health promotion

Let us examine the issues a stage further by exploring the activities of health education and ill-health prevention in more detail. If you refer back to your list of health promotion you consider you had been exposed to (Exercise 8.4), you may have included a variety of approaches, some telling you what to do, some increasing your knowledge about health options. There are several models of health education. Although some have overlapping aims, we will attempt to distinguish them according to:

- the overall goal guiding the model;

- whether it is the professional or the client who sets the agenda.

Medical model/negative health model

Health education based on this model usually has a single disease or disability or a group of them as its focus. It's concerned with:

- informing people, e.g., about the dangers of smoking in relation to lung and heart disease.
- high risk individuals taking up screening services, e.g., for HIV, high cholesterol, breast cancer.
- add an example below relevant to your particular area of interest:
- _____

In this type of health education professionals take on the role of expert adviser or information giver. Communication tends to be in one direction only, that is from the professional to a client or patient.

The impetus for developing this type of health education programme may be a high incidence of a particular disease. A useful exercise would be to identify national and/or local health education campaigns in your area and try to identify why they were developed at a particular time and find out whether they were successful.

Behaviour change or modification model

This approach focuses on encouraging individuals to change their behaviour to increase their chances of avoiding ill health or of developing a better level of health. It usually focuses on the adoption of a healthy lifestyle. We are bombarded with messages coming from this approach, e.g. stop smoking, drink in moderation, practise safe sex, eat low fat/high fibre diets. Some people may feel they are being 'told' what to do and that they are at fault if they do not follow the advice – does this sound familiar in relation to smoking? This approach appears to have two underlying assumptions: that health status is determined by individual behaviour, and that individuals can choose to change their behaviour, _and_ have the resources to do so, if they are advised of the healthy alternatives. We'll explore this idea in more detail later but think back to the WHO definition of health promotion we looked at earlier. This emphasized health promotion, and enabling people to take healthy options, which requires more than information or advice giving.

Informed choice model

This approach is more concerned with increasing knowledge and understanding so that individuals can make the most appropriate choice for their situation, often referred to as an informed choice. Although there appears to be more partnership with the client in this approach, it is usually the professional or State who chooses which subject will be addressed. For example, it may be the national school curriculum or the school governors who decide if sexual health education will be part of school education.

There's an assumption here that everyone has equal opportunities to make an informed choice. We'll return to this issue later.

Client-focused model

The ownership of the interaction is much more with the client. This approach should be responsive to what the client wants to know or consider. The client, not the health professional, sets the agenda. This approach has much in common with community development approaches to care. It sounds good and appears to avoid some of the pitfalls we've identified in the other models. It means that the client's priorities, interests and concerns are addressed, but we have not found perfection, there are still some potential problems. An important point to consider is 'Do we always know what we need to know'? Is it fair to leave agenda setting solely to the client, what about those issues they are unaware of or choose to avoid, what should be done about them?

Collective or societal model

This model moves away from the individual level and takes on a societal approach to health education/prevention/promotion. It may involve political or legislative issues, e.g., seatbelt use or the provision of cycle paths. As a consequence of this model it may be easier for individuals to choose the healthy option or to fulfil their health potential with e.g., provision of leisure facilities, subsidized rates for leisure facilities or it may enhance the population's chances of not encountering a negative health risk and so increase their chances of being able to pursue a healthy lifestyle. This model generally operates on a longer time scale to the other models we've discussed. This type of health promotion is often imposed rather than chosen through, for example, smoking bans.

The type of actions people working with this model might take include:

- protecting in a preventative way, e.g., provision of clean water supply; supplementing certain food with extra minerals and vitamins.
- protecting in an educative way – this could be directed towards policy-makers lobbying politicians or service providers for a particular service or legislation; it could also relate to general dissemination to the public about a health care issue, e.g., the mass education and publicity campaign associated with HIV or action to prevent 'cot death' campaigns.
- protecting against negative health effects through, e.g., legislation regarding levels of lead emissions from car exhausts.

Exercise 8.5

Identify another couple of examples of the collective approach to health promotion:

_____

_____

_____

_____

_____

To consider how these different models might apply to some specific health issues work through Exercise 8.6.

Exercise 8.6

Using the table below consider which of these models might be useful (several may be used to varying time scales) to address the health issues from varying perspectives. There are a couple of blank spaces to use with your own examples.

	Medical model	Behaviour change	Informed choice	Client-focused	Collective or societal
Smoking:					
Diet:					
HIV:					
Accident prevention:					
Stress management:					
Ability to deal with personal development:					
Adolescence/ageing:					
Controlling car exhaust emissions:					
Personal confidence building:					

Why do people not act on health promotion information or advice?

We've just identified a wide range of health-promoting activities that we may meet as part of our everyday life. It seems appropriate to ask therefore why there are large numbers of people who do not achieve their health potential. Why do people not follow this widely available advice and take up the services on offer that could possibly enhance their health status? First of all, let's focus on you. Work through Exercise 8.7 (overleaf).

One reason you might have identified in Exercise 8.7 is that everyone is not immediately receptive to, for example, health education. Giving a 'healthy message' is not always the most appropriate starting point. Often people need to be motivated and empowered to actually consider their health before they can begin to think about making some commitment to promote their health. People need to consider their health is important, believe that they can improve it, believe that they have options. Clients may need to be helped to raise their self-esteem or feelings of self-worth in order to have the confidence to set their own agenda and be active participants in the health-promoting process. We are really talking about empowerment of individuals or communities, a key feature of the enabling process referred to earlier

In order to try to answer these questions we need to ponder another set of questions about the health promotion intervention:

- Is the health promotion intervention provided in the most appropriate and effective way, is it suitable for the person/s concerned?

Exercise 8.7

It's fairly safe to assume that you have considerable knowledge about what is healthy lifestyle practice in relation to diet, alcohol consumption, exercise, etc., but have you modified your behaviour in line with your knowledge? Make a list of health advice you know but do not follow and try to identify the reasons.

What about other people, such as clients, patients or family and friends? Try to identify reasons why they do or do not follow the various publicized advice on health.

- Is the health promotion intervention provided in the most appropriate place?
- Is the health promotion intervention delivered using the most acceptable and appropriate resources?

Let's consider these questions in turn.

Is the health promotion intervention provided in the most appropriate and effective format, is it suitable for the person/s concerned?

The first important fact to remember with respect to health promotion interventions is 'one size does not fit all'. Health promotion interventions need to be planned in response to assessed needs. The provider must have a good understanding of why certain individuals or populations make particular health choices. Is the intervention based on the reality of people's lives? This last sentiment is central to the UK government's 2004 public health policy *Choosing Health: Making Healthy Choices Easier.* To quote from the document:

'Traditional methods of improving health are becoming outdated and new approaches and new action are needed to secure progress' (p. 9). Exercise 8.8 (facing) provides you with an opportunity to put this into practice.

Turn your mind to television advertising for a moment – think of a well-known product – reflect on how the advertising of that product has changed over the past 20 years. Perhaps it is a lesson we can transfer to health promotion. Indeed, social marketing principles are increasingly being considered in relation to health promotion. Beishon (2005) lists the four 'Ps' on which social marketing is based:

- *Product* – 'ensuring a product or service suits the target market'.

Exercise 8.8

Identify two health promotion situations or interventions that you have utilized recently:

1

2

Ok – this is your opportunity to show how innovative you can be: address the health promotion issues you have identified above, but in new ways . . .

- *Price* – 'understanding what people feel they have to give up to benefit'.
- *Place* – 'ensuring the product is accessible and usable by the target audience'.
- *Promotion* – 'letting people know that what is on offer is worth having'.

Look back at Exercise 8.8 and consider whether product, place, price and promotion issues were addressed.

Let's move on to the second of the three questions listed above.

Is the health promotion intervention provided in the most appropriate place?

The setting or location for health promotion needs to be considered for a number of reasons:

- The setting may generate particular health promotion needs. For example, compare carrying out health promotion in a university, a primary school, a factory, a sheltered housing complex. How might levels of health literacy differ, how might population cohesiveness differ?
- Settings provide access to certain populations who may otherwise be difficult to access or who may not seek out health promotion, for example, male factory workers.
- Review of the setting may provide measures to impact on the individual health choices, for example, the removal of a soft drinks vending machine from a school.
- Health and health promotion may become part of the agenda for that setting.
- Consideration of the setting is essential to fully understand the needs and potential responses to those needs – remember the issues of locating health promotion in the reality of people's lives.

Now let's address the third question.

Is the health promotion intervention delivered using the most acceptable and appropriate resources?

Do health promoters make sufficient use of electronic information sources? Have health promoters changed their approach in response to the vast amount of health related information available through the Internet? Could we make us of email communication to remind people about a health promotion message or to provide support during the implementation of a new health choice? Do we limit our health promotion activity to getting people to the point of deciding to change their health choices, but then fail to provide any support to maintain the activity? Must the professional always be the provider? For example, are alternatives such as peer educators given adequate consideration?

How do we know if health promotion interventions are being effective?

The first issue we have to consider is, what would success look like?

- people attend a health promotion activity;
- people consider their health choices, but do not make any changes;
- people consider their health choices and make a change;
- people feel better about themselves and their communities;
- morbidity levels reduce;
- mortality levels reduce.

Any of these changes would be an acceptable indicator of success – depending on the aim of the health promotion intervention. Giving sufficient thought to the aim is often a neglected aspect of health promotion practice. It is not uncommon to hear health promoters stating a very broad aim such as a reduction in coronary heart disease. However, this is really not an adequate aim:

- The reduction, if it occurred, would not be immediately apparent – it could be 20 years hence. Is it reasonable to continue a health promotion intervention all that time assuming and hoping that it will lead to the desired effect?
- This health promotion activity will probably be one of several that the client/s will be exposed to – how do you know that your intervention is making an effective contribution?

It is important therefore that health promoters articulate the short-, medium- and long-term steps to the ultimate goal so that ongoing, staged evaluation can occur.

Reflecting back on earlier discussions about locating health promotion in the reality of people's lives means that evaluation cannot be a generic activity. Have you ever experienced a health promotion intervention being successful with one group and then experience a disappointing outcome when you try again with another group? This raises the importance of recognizing the impact of a particular context on the health promotion outcome.

How broad is the scope of health promotion?

We have focused largely on the individual level, but health promotion is much wider than individual issues and individual actions. It is concerned with global warming, food preservation, crop production, engineering investment to achieve less pollution, transport policies, allocation of resources to different sectors of health care services. The message is health promotion combines a wide number of issues which complement each other to assist with the achievement of better levels of health. Some will have as their focus preventing ill health, some the protection and maintenance of current health levels, others on attempting to achieve higher levels of health for individuals and also on reducing the variation in health status across populations.

The impact of any action or policy aimed at promoting health can often be limited if it is only focused on one perspective. Health is a multi-factoral concept, actions that include several routes to achieving the aim of promoting health are often more successful. Use Exercise 8.9 to help you think through some of the many ways that public policy can influence health.

Exercise 8.9

Identify some national policy changes in your country over the last ten years and consider their impact on health. You may wish to consider such things as transport and road policy, changes to the organization of health care, changes in education, policies towards the unemployed and so on.

Conclusion: so, what is health promotion?

Let's return to our original question – 'What is health promotion'? We might now want to think of it as:

- an umbrella term whose facets include ill health prevention activities, health education and health protection, but whose aim is achieving the highest potential levels of health and not merely avoiding ill health;
- an activity that incorporates prevention, education and protection.

Client participation in health promotion activities may be of varying types:

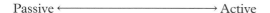

Passive ←————————————————→ Active

Participation may be the individual's choice or they may need to be assisted or empowered to participate.

Finally, health promoting actions may be taken at an individual or collective level. A collective level could be on a world-wide perspective.

Summary

Write your own summary of this chapter by addressing the following questions.

1   Write a short paragraph to distinguish between the activities of health education, health protection and health promotion.

2   Briefly describe the key features of the five models of health education.

3   Write a short paragraph which summarizes how you see yourself, as a health care professional, being involved in health promotion (either now or in the future).

Now reflect again on what your skills and knowledge currently are, where there are gaps and any actions arising.

Public health standards	
Surveillance & assessment	
Promoting & protecting	
Developing quality & risk management	
Collaborative working for health	
Developing programmes & services & reducing inequalities	
Policy & strategy development & implementation	
Working with & for communities	
Strategic leadership	
Research & Development	
Ethically managing self, people & resources	

9

Health needs analysis

What is a health need?

How can we identify what are the health needs of a particular community?

How do health needs differ between groups and localities and over time?

How can health needs analysis be used to design policies and action plans aimed to improve health?

What is the contribution of health impact assessment to health needs analysis?

After working through this chapter you should be able to:

- define different types of need;
- identify different units for the analysis of health needs;
- list the functions of a community health need analysis;
- describe a framework for the process of community health profiling and health needs analysis;
- list possible sources of data which can be used to inform the profiling process;
- use health needs analysis to design action plans for health improvement;
- describe the contribution of health impact assessment to health improvement.

What is involved in 'health needs' analysis?

Several concepts and activities are involved in analysing health needs. There are at least five issues for consideration:

- what definition or interpretation of 'health' we are using;
- what is a health need;
- what kind of information we need to undertake a health needs analysis;
- where we access the data to provide the information;
- how we use the analysis to plan for health improvement.

Both health and need are not absolute concepts, but are relative to the time and people concerned. Between individuals, groups, regions and countries there will be differing definitions and prioritization of health and what represents a genuine health need. As our expectations of health, and our cultural traditions of the role of the family and the state and the health and social care availability vary, so will our definitions of health and health need.

What is health?

There are many definitions of health, but it will suffice for this discussion to say that health has physical, social and psychological components and it is not a static but a dynamic concept. Although we will look at the idea of need and health need in more detail later, let's use the health need idea to further explore the question of what is health. We will do this by working through Exercise 9.1.

Exercise 9.1

Consider the following statements:

A – A health need exists when health is absent.
B – No matter how healthy you are, everyone has health needs.
C – Health needs can be predicted by factors such as age, gender and social position.
D – If you are unaware of your health need, that means it must not be important.
E – Personal health needs are different to population health needs.

Which do you agree with: A, B, C, D or E?

Compare your responses in Exercise 9.1 with the following comments about each of the statements in Exercise 9.1 and the related service aims and limitations:

A   This represents a fairly narrow view of health, i.e., health is the absence of disease. If we accepted this view, our aim would be limited to avoidance of ill health. Are you aware of any such services? What about health in terms of well-being and achieving individual health potential?; these dimensions of health are missing in this response.

B   This is probably the nearest to the truth. All individuals have health needs, either to maintain health or to improve their level of health. Service provision therefore needs to cover a wide continuum from health maintenance, protection and improvement to treatments and care for ill health

C   This is a rather impractical statement at the individual level, though relevant at the population level. It is true to say, for example, that many women might benefit from certain intervention programmes, such as cervical screening, that children will benefit from immunization programmes. However, it does not acknowledge that the approach to health needs has to be both dynamic and individual. In doing this, it does not acknowledge the need for and skills in health needs analysis beyond that of a very generic population approach, i.e., all children, all females.

D   This statement doesn't really hold water. Unless you have knowledge of your health need you can't make an informed choice of whether to act on them or not. Health needs analysis has an important role in assessing population health knowledge status and action planning to develop health literacy.

E   The answer to this statement is, 'Yes and no!' Personal health needs may overlap with population needs or they may differ. Population needs often take account of the greatest good for the greatest number of people.

Let us explore the issue of need in more detail.

What is a need?

Let's think about how we become aware that we have a need. This will help us to develop our definition of the word. Start by working through Exercise 9.2.

Exercise 9.2

Think about any need(s) you have had recently, possibly but not necessarily related to health. List them below.

Next to each one describe how you came to identify it as a need, e.g., was it based on specialist advice, on something you read, on peer group pressure, on feeling unwell, and so on?

Your responses for Exercise 9.2 probably indicated several different ways of identifying needs. Let's identify some of these by considering some possible responses to the question, 'What needs might I have in relation to my car?'

1   The car has recently had an MOT and the mechanic told me that the exhaust must be replaced.

2   The car exhaust is becoming noisy and I think it will have to be replaced shortly.

3   The car manufacturer recommends renewing the exhaust after 50,000 kilometres so I will book the car into the garage.

4   My friend has the same age car as mine and has had to have the exhaust replaced, so mine will probably need replacing soon as well.

Now let's try to analyse these responses:

1   Someone makes you aware of a need you had not actually identified yourself.

2   You may be aware of a need yourself and may or may not do something about it. Have you ever had toothache, but not gone to the dentist!

3   You know you have a need and take action to address it.

4   You may only become aware of a need if you compare your situation with someone else.

Let's now try and relate this discussion about need to health. We look at four levels of health need that were first identified by Bradshaw (1972). Each type of need is listed below with examples, together with a space to allow you to add an example or examples of your own.

NORMATIVE NEED: what the expert or professional defines as a need.
Example: the medical definition of overweight and obesity
Provide your own example:

FELT NEED: a need that can be equated with a want.
Example: the desire to lose weight
Provide your own example:

EXPRESSED NEED: a need or want that is translated into action.
Example: seeking advice about weight reduction
Provide your own example:

COMPARATIVE NEED: need identified comparing the services received by one group of individuals with those received by a similar group.
Example: group for whom no weight-reducing treatment is available compared to a similar group who has a service
Provide your own example:

You will have realized that the situation can become very complex very quickly. This is particularly the case when there is a lack of awareness or a disagreement between the parties involved in defining a health need. This could be professional and client, client and client, client and government policy-maker, social worker and nurse, doctor and health visitor. For example, someone may desire to lose weight when from a medical point of view his/her weight is perfectly normal; a group may demand access to a particular weight-reducing treatment because the service is available elsewhere, but there may be no evidence that the treatment does any good. This latter example illustrates that the problem not only lies with the identification of need but on deciding when a need has been met. We return again to the problem of, how do we measure health?

Measurements of health

There are many different approaches to measuring health, reflecting that health is a multidimensional concept. One of the commonest approaches is to use mortality data, that is death rates. Or where they exist, morbidity, that is illness rates for specific diseases (see also Chapters 2 and 3). Another way to measure health by proxy is to measure the level of certain lifestyle behaviours in the population. The British government's national targets in 2005 included considerations of mortality, morbidity and lifestyle measures:

- to reduce mortality rates from heart disease and stroke by at least 40 per cent in people under 75 by 2010;
- to halt the year-on-year rise in obesity among children under 11 by 2010;
- to reduce adult smoking rates to 21 per cent or less by 2010.

These types of targets represent limited measurements of health. What they do not give us is any indication of how the health need is perceived.

Exercise 9.3

Review the health targets set out in your government policies to identify what types of data are used and how health need is perceived. It would also be useful to look at documents from a few years ago to identify any changes.

An example of a different approach is that taken by Townsend et al. (1988) in their study of health and deprivation. Rather than using specific diseases, i.e., stroke or suicide, they used the following dimensions of health:

- death registrations;
- birth weight indicators;
- permanent sickness rates.

They combined these to form an 'Overall Health Index' and because they acknowledged that health is affected by social circumstances, they also developed a deprivation index using census information on unemployment, car ownership, home
ownership and overcrowding. Some data following this approach for health districts
in the north east of England are shown in Exercise 9.4. Look at this now.

Exercise 9.4

Look at the table, then consider the question below it.

District	Health score	Deprivation score
Hartlepool	3.25	2.02
North Tees	1.60	−1.67
South Tees	0.70	0.96
Northumberland	−3.94	−3.25
Gateshead	2.59	3.73
Newcastle	1.59	3.70
North Tyneside	0.64	0.41
Sunderland	0.27	3.73

Note: The higher scores indicate greater ill health and deprivation.

What inferences can you draw from this chart about the relationship between social
circumstances and health status?

In your response to Exercise 9.4 you may have included some of the following
comments:

1   It appears that health and the level of deprivation may be linked:
    - Northumberland appears to have high levels of health and low levels of
      deprivation.
    - North Tyneside appears to have a slightly higher than average level of
      deprivation and a less than average health status.
2   The correlation between deprivation and health scores is not consistent:
    - Hartlepool's health score is rather worse than the deprivation score.
3   Some areas appear to have a health score better than expected, in view of the
    deprivation score:
    - Sunderland's health score is just below average but the deprivation score is
      considerably below average.

In order to make more sense of these scores, we would need to know more about each area, such as how the population responds to deprivation and whether deprivation has been long-term or a recent event. We would also need to investigate how well these scores actually reflect the health and social circumstances of the people living in those districts. Tools to assist in further exploring and measuring other dimensions of health and factors potentially influencing health are now being developed. One example would be the Health Poverty Index (see Further reading).

Another aspect of health that we can attempt to measure is social capital. The Health Development Agency (2004) describe this as comprising:

- social resources – informal arrangements between neighbours or within a faith community;
- collective resources – self-help groups, credit unions, community safety schemes;
- economic resources – levels of employment, access to green, open spaces;
- cultural resources – libraries, art centres, local schools.

One measurement tool in the UK is the General Household Survey response to questions on trust and reciprocity, social networks and civic engagement.

So far we have examined definitions of health and need and very briefly touched on the measurement of health. We need to put these issues together to consider health needs analysis.

Health needs analysis

Health needs analysis can be carried out from multiple levels and perspectives. This is illustrated in Figure 9.1. Let's work through some of the issues surrounding health needs analysis from different perspectives. Before we can embark on any analysis process, we need to be aware of the overall goal of the process that will guide the process in both a qualitative and quantative manner. Look at Exercise 9.5.

Exercise 9.5

Consider the following goals. Think through the type of analysis processes you might use to help you achieve, and know whether you have achieved, each of these goals:

• To reduce deaths from coronary heart disease by 15 percent by the year 2010.

• To reduce the number of children with dental caries by 10 percent by the year 2015.

• To add years to life and life to years.

• To provide a service that is responsive to the demands of the users of the service.

DEFINITION OF HEALTH

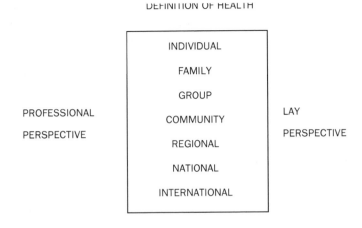

OVERALL GOAL

Figure 9.1 Levels and perspectives in health needs assessments

The first two goals in Exercise 9.5 are to do with mortality and morbidity respectively from medically defined diseases. Health needs analysis to assist in the achievement of these goals might concentrate on rates of these conditions and identified risk factors for them. The third goal refers not to only adding years to life but also to 'add life to years'. This could be interpreted simply in terms of reducing the prevalence of disease in older age, or might be interpreted more broadly and positively in terms of adding to the quality of life in other ways as well. Clearly which interpretation is used will make a big difference as to how 'health needs' are defined and analysed. Finally, assessing health needs with the aim of providing a more client-orientated service will mean that we need to find out what the client wants, what they think of the current service, and so on. None of these approaches are mutually exclusive. The point is that the type of information required depends upon what it is we want to achieve. The more levels that are included, the more comprehensive the health needs analysis.

There are many examples of health needs analysis carried out at different levels internationally, nationally, regionally and at community level. Some examples include:

- International – World Health Organization, *Health for All in the 21st Century.*
- National – In England an example is the Department of Health, *Choosing Health* 2004, targets for specific health problems such as to reduce the death rate from suicide and undetermined injury by at least 20 per cent by 2010. Can you identify equivalent documents produced by other countries?
- Regional – Phillimore and Beattie's (1994) epidemiological study of the northern region of England 1981–91 would be one example. Another would be *Taking Measures* (HDA 2004b) analysis of alcohol misuse in the north-west of England. Can you identify an example from the region in which you work?

- Community – an example would be the HNA that Primary Care Trusts in England are obliged to conduct on which to base their health plans (Department of Health 2001). Can you identify a copy of the latest health plan produced by your Primary Care Trust (it may be available via their web page) or whatever body is responsible for analysing and planning health service provision at a local level?

Such analyses are used to inform policies impacting on health and to set priorities for action. A tailoring process needs to occur – national policies need to be made appropriate to local needs, systems and structures. How do they do this? It would be virtually impossible to make an individual health needs analysis on all of the population and one would have to question if it were really necessary or whether intermediate levels between nation and individual level would be most appropriate. A number of approaches have been taken. The levels at which health needs analysis are done often reflect the administrative units for the provision of social and health services. The health needs analysis can then serve the purpose of guiding the provision of the health and social services in that area.

An advantage of using such administrative units is that many statistics, such as census information and mortality rates are published for those areas. A disadvantage is that the units may not equate with what the population considers to be a 'natural' community and may contain very diverse populations living under very different circumstances. Another option is to base a health needs analysis on a neighbourhood or community. Let's explore this type of unit of analysis, which is made up of a number of components. We need to consider a five-step process:

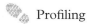 Profiling

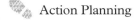 Analysis and prioritizing

Action Planning

Implementation

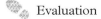 Evaluation

Community health profiling

Again we need to consider some of the components of the idea before we look at the process. How can we identify a community? Can we set boundaries from a map? Is it determined by the organization of primary health care services? By the schools the children attend? Can it actually be described in geographical terms or must it also have a subjective element of belonging? Consider some of these issues for yourself by working through Exercise 9.6.

Exercise 9.6

Think about yourself: list the community or communities you belong to.

For each one give the reasons why you consider yourself a member of that community.

There are many possibilities you may have considered in Exercise 9.6.

- The housing estate. Two housing estates could be situated very close, but dependent on the different types of housing, the inhabitants may see themselves as belonging to one community spread over two estates or to two different communities.
- The area of the town in which you live. This may be the east or west part of a town or the inner city or the suburbs, etc.
- Geographical boundaries. Communities may be determined by the presence of a river, major road network, etc.
- Your place of work and/or job. You may consider that you belong to two communities, your place of work and your home, or they may be part of the same community, particularly if you live near your work and many of your neighbours work at the same place.
- Your religious group and/or your place of worship.
- Your ethnic group. It may be that you consider yourself part of a wider community embracing all members of your ethnic group across an area, or just the people of the same ethnic group in your immediate area.
- Your age group, such as 20s, over-40s etc.
- Your civil state, e.g., married with children, married without children, single parent, single without children, etc.
- Your sexual orientation.
- Your political beliefs and activities.
- And so on . . .

Now that we have identified what might be a 'community', we need to consider why we might want to profile it.

Why profile community health?

Although general levels of health have improved over the years, there is still plenty of room for further development. There is a wide variation in the levels of health achieved in different communities, e.g., rural, inner city, by socio-economic status.

Such variations are vividly described in an example of health variations in the UK presented in *Choosing Health* (Department of Health 2004: 78) that is adapted below.

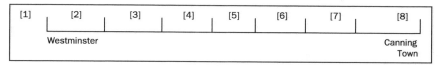

Figure 9.2 London Underground tube stations

Source: Adapted from *Choosing Health*, (Department of Health 2004: 78).

Station [8], Canning Town is approximately 8 miles east of station [1] Westminster and the journey involves a total of eight tube stations. That is geographically a small area but there is considerable variability in life expectancy within it. In fact, for each tube station travelled east, nearly one year of life expectancy is lost.

The desire to tackle such health inequalities has led to an increase in public health and inter-sectoral approaches to health and social care. The public health agenda is prominent in many government policies where proactive approaches are emphasized. New kinds of working in a multi-sectoral way that reflects a broad definition of health have resulted in the development of area-based initiatives and in regeneration activities (Russel and Killoran 2000). Simply stated, there is dissatisfaction with a reliance on a reactive approach to health care that emphasizes dealing with problems and issues when they arise rather than trying to anticipate and respond to them at an earlier stage. There is increasing support in many government policies (see Further reading) for a change in approach, to one that is more proactive in identifying locality health needs and responding specifically to them. Health needs analysis enables the identification of needs specific to a particular population so that service development and provision can be needs-responsive. This in turn fits well with the growing need to be cognizant of the effective use of resources. There is international interest in attempting to quantify and measure the impact of services aimed at improving health.

Let us think next of some of the ways in which the local community/area in which you live can affect your health. Consider this in Exercise 9.7.

Exercise 9.7

List the ways in which you feel the area community/area in which you live has, or could have, an influence on your health (list positive and negative influences).

Depending on your particular community and the perspective you have adopted you may have highlighted some of the following:

- Employment availability, together with easy access to work and/or major services.
- Adequacy and accessibility of services such as health, education, social services.

- Appropriateness and quality of housing to suit your needs.
- People around for support and social contact.
- Levels of crime/vandalism, and how safe you feel.
- Accessibility of recreational activities.
- Transport facilities and networks.
- The pleasantness and quality of the local environment or the stigma attached to your local environment.

The community in which you live can obviously have a significant influence on your health and profiling the community may therefore highlight health needs. The needs identified by profiles may serve several functions. For example, a profile can increase understanding/knowledge of an area in order to make an objective and systematic health needs analysis in order to effectively translate national targets for local application. This systematic approach also avoids reliance on preconceived ideas. People are often guilty of making assumptions, such as that an affluent area will not have a problem with child abuse, whereas we appear to be more ready to acknowledge the possibility of its existence in a more deprived area, or that only mothers at the higher end of the social scale will breast feed. However, in reality such broad generalizations are not true. As with all health care interventions, a systematic assessment of needs is essential. The clear message here is that an objective search for health needs has to be performed. This should be done in partnership with the population because of the relative definitions of need and health that the professional and layperson may hold and the viability of any resulting action plan.

We have identified how the community can affect health and the purposes of a community health needs assessment, we now need to explore how to actually profile a community and consider how we analyse health needs.

The process of community health profiling

As we have already identified, health needs analysis and community profiling may be carried out for different reasons. It is impossible to give a standard format for the process and number of templates are available (see Further reading section). There are certain key issues that will always need to be addressed, although the emphasis will vary. Amassing data about an area is only the first stage in a health needs analysis and certainly not the full story.

A profiling framework is presented in Table 9.1, identifying key factors in the community that may influence health in a positive or negative way. Being too prescriptive with respect to a profiling tool defeats the purpose of the exercise. This particular framework may not be the most suitable tool to use to profile in all communities. However, it is possible to adapt the framework by, for example, supplementing headings that are particularly applicable to an area and then making an estimation of the resources and deficits in a particular community.

An important component of community profiling is that the population being profiled must be involved in the process. This helps to avoid only identifying overt

Table 9.1 A framework for community profiling

Factor	Positive or negative resource	Indicators
Environment		Local industry, maps, accident rates, crime/vandalism
Housing		Observation, local authority, housing associations, homeless figures, hostels
Demography		Census data, caseload profiles, practice profiles
Social class		Employment, lifestyle, values, access to car
Transport		Car ownership, public transport, costs
Shops		Range of goods, price levels, accessibility
Religious groups		Types, location, attendance, resources
Leisure facilities		Recreation facilities, pubs, restaurants, accessibility, subsidization, sports teams, scout groups, parks
Education		Pre-school, school, adult, location, cost, range of levels
Health care		Hospital and primary care, location, accessibility, patient participation, alternative therapies, user representation opportunities, waiting lists, level of care fro the population
Voluntary		Faith-based groups, support groups, self-help groups
Character		History, warmth, friendliness, style, design, cohesion, social capital
Family structures		Mobile population, single parents, lone elderly, working parents
Economics		Unemployment level, overcrowding, affluence, poverty

needs or needs generated by the professional or service providers who have their own agendas. This is in keeping with the general policy drive to increase public and patient participation in health care (see Further reading). The workers carrying out the profile therefore engage the local population in the process. This necessitates being familiar with the community and being able to identify local sources of information to develop the profile in partnership (see Further reading). Community participation has mainly developed since the 1950s. It incorporates aspects of four theoretical constructs; community development, people's participation, empowerment and action research (HDA 2000). A participatory appraisal approach offers a means of surveying the population in a way that allows high levels of participation in a time-efficient manner. Qualitative methods that may be used in the process include focus groups, and message boards in local venues such as shopping centres or schools. Visualization tools such as drawing are also used to widen communication from the written or spoken word. (see Further reading). The data collection process is taken to the population and so provides opportunities to access the views of those people who may not otherwise take part in a survey of health needs.

Exercise 9.8

Identify venues for undertaking participatory appraisal and which particular appraisal strategies you could employ.

Think about the needs of different age groups, non-English speakers, and people with low reading ages.

Identifying the resources of an area is only one part of a community health profile. As mentioned earlier, it is not just about amassing information about an area and the populations living or working there. The profiler must have the knowledge and skill to make an assessment of the health needs of the area based on the information gathered and on routinely available local and national data, such as:

- census information;
- mortality rates;
- birth rates;
- morbidity data;
- service utilization, i.e., immunization rates, smear take-up rates;
- national patterns of demography;
- information on society values and changes in family life structure;
- government policy on pollution, housing, benefit levels, community care.

All these issues must be considered within a knowledge base of health determinants and health impact.

What happens after profiling?

The next stage in the process is undertaking an analysis of health need. This is achieved by answering questions such as:

- What resources does this community have?
- What resources does this community lack?
- What are the health needs as perceived by different lay and professional groups?
- What is the health status of this population in comparison with nationally set targets?
- Are there specific areas for improvement?
- Are there clear priorities or multiple competing issues?
- Is there a consensus on priorities?
- Has there been any changes since the last health needs analysis or health impact assessment plan?

Exercise 9.9

Add any more questions to ask of the data:

Ideally all stakeholders involved in the potential response and all those who will be affected by the response to the HNA should be involved in this stage of the process. One example across sector collaborations would be a Health Partnership Board (see Further reading).

Exercise 9.10

Think of strategies you could use to involve the population and multiple agencies in this analysis process in your area.

The next stage in the process is prioritizing the agenda for action. This will involve addressing a number of questions:

- Are there needs that require urgent attention?
- Are there some needs, which although important, could be identified for action in the future?
- Is there a recognized solution or intervention to an identified need?
- Is there agreement between stakeholders about priority setting?
- Are there any budgetary or funding restrictions on what action can be planned?
- Have the needs changed since the previous HNA? Why? Have previous action plans been successful in effectively meeting a health need? How can sustainability be managed? Can other needs now be prioritized?

- Are the needs the same as those identified the previous HNA? Why? Have the interventions been unsuccessful – can alternatives be identified?
- Are health needs similar or different from neighboring areas? And why might that be?

An action plan to meet the identified needs is the next level of activity. This is an appropriate time to consider introducing health impact assessment (HIA) into the process. The Health Development Agency (2002: ii) defines HIA as 'an approach that can help identify and consider the health and inequalities impacts of a proposal on a given population'. It can be a prospective activity, carried out in the planning stages of a proposal. Alternatively it can be retrospective, identifying the impact of an implemented proposal on a population. A prospective approach is economically and ethically preferable. Details of the process can be found in the further reading section of this chapter. A brief example is provided below to begin to clarify the process involved. Blank spaces are left for you to add other potential issues.

Exercise 9.11

Plans have been submitted to build a small shopping centre near to a new housing development. Potential positive and negative health impacts could be identified to aid the decision making process

---

POSITIVE

Impact on determinants of health

- The shopping centre would provide a venue for social contact and a community focus.
- The shops would provide employment opportunities.
- Increased access to food products.

- _____

- _____

Consequences

- Potential for social isolation may be reduced and social cohesion enhanced.
- Employed people generally have better health status.
- Facilitates opportunities for healthy diet consumption.

- _____

- _____

NEGATIVE

Impact on determinants of health

- Increased traffic in the area.

- _____

- _____

Consequences

- Increased pollution, increased risk of accidents.

- _____

- _____

It may be possible to control for negative consequences. In the example above, appropriate road safety measure could deal with a potential negative impact of a shopping centre development.

The action plan will then be implemented. Evaluation of impact measures also need to be included in order to monitor effectiveness. This should include consideration of short-term, long-term and cumulative changes.

Summary

Respond to questions below and complete your own summary of this chapter.

1   Health needs analysis is a dynamic process that may be undertaken at an individual, community and national level. Give an example of an assessment carried out at these different levels.
    - Individual:
    - Community:
    - National:

2   There are different types of acknowledged and unacknowledged need and there may be differences between professional and lay opinions.

    List four types of need and give an example of each that relates specifically to your area of health or social care.

    •

    •

    •

    •

3   The community (used here in the sense of the area in which one lives) can have significant influences on health.

    Give three examples of how a community an affect health positively and three examples of how it could have a negative effect on health.

    Positive:

    •

    •

    •

Negative:

-

-

-

4   Profiling involves the systematic collection of data.

List six sources of data that would inform the profiling process. Include both qualitative and quantitative sources:

-

-

-

-

-

-

5   In order to complete a health needs analysis for a whole community, it may be necessary to apply this framework to several groups within the community in order to come up with an overall health needs analysis and priorities for action. Consider this list of possible residents:

- active elderly lady, caring for her husband who suffers with dementia;
- young mother with two children under 5;
- adolescent from a household living in poverty;
- single, employed, 40-year-old woman;
- recently retired couple;
- a young adult with a learning disability, living with his/her family.

Using a community you are familiar with, such as an area you are studying, or living in or working in:

- Apply the profiling framework from the point of view of three of the individual case histories presented above.
- Indicate how and from where you would access the necessary data.

A blank profiling framework is provided (Table 9.2) which could be photocopied for further use.

Table 9.2 Blank community profiling framework

Factors	Positive or negative resource	Indicators
Environment		
Housing		
Demography		
Social class		
Transport		
Shops		
Religious groups		
Leisure facilities		
Education		
Health care		
Voluntary		
Character		
Family structures		
Economics		

Now reflect again on what your skills and knowledge currently are, where there are gaps and any actions arising.

Public health standards	
Surveillance & assessment	
Promoting & protecting	
Developing quality & risk management	
Collaborative working for health	
Developing programmes & services & reducing inequalities	
Policy & strategy development & implementation	
Working with & for communities	
Strategic leadership	
Research & Development	
Ethically managing self, people & resources	

10

Principles of screening

What do we mean by 'screening'?

Why screen for one disease and not another?

How are decisions made about who will benefit from the screening?

Do those at risk always take up the screening on offer?

After working through this chapter you should be able to:

- define screening and understand how it differs from surveillance or case identification;
- identify different types of screening and the rationale for their selection;
- understand how the population who will benefit from screening are identified;
- list the criteria or principles for a screening programme;
- be aware of some of the factors that may influence the uptake of available screening.

What is screening?

What do we mean by the term 'screening'? What's the purpose of developing and implementing screening programmes? Screening is in essence about looking for health problems, but if not planned and carried out correctly, it can be an ineffective, inappropriate and unethical attempt at health care. We firstly need to clarify exactly what we mean by the term screening.

Screening is a commonly, although sometimes imprecisely, used term. By comparing and contrasting it with some other health care activities, it is possible to identify its key components.

Do this in Exercise 10.1.

Exercise 10.1

Consider the following statements:

A   Screening is a diagnostic activity.
B   Screening is an identification process.
C   Screening is about identifying disease at an early stage.
D   Screening is concerned with health status improvement for the individual.

Which statement(s) most accurately describe screening: A, B, C or D?

A   Screening may identify someone who needs to be referred in order for a diagnosis. Screening is not a substitute for diagnosis, it is a different and distinct activity.

B   This is a good description of screening, a process of identifying those at risk to some health status threat. Diagnosis to establish the existence of disease or precursor to a disease should follow.

C   Screening is indeed about identifying disease at an early stage so that treatment can be instigated and the prognosis improved. However, screening is also used to identify individuals at risk from developing a disease some time in the future so that preventative action can take place to prevent the occurrence of the problem.

D   It is true to say that screening is carried out for individual benefit but that is only part of the story. Screening also has a role in the control of infectious disease in that it can be used to identify the carrier of a disease in the community, i.e., tuberculosis, food poisoning, resistant staphylococcus wound infection. Screening is often established on the basis of whether it will improve the health of the population.

These issues are well summed up in this definition of screening:

> The presumptive identification of unrecognised disease or defect by the application of tests, examinations or other procedures which can be applied rapidly. Screening tests sort out the apparently well persons who probably have a disease from those who probably do not.
>
> (Last and Spasoff 2000: 118)

Screening can fulfil a number of functions. Review of a number of screening programmes in the United Kingdom identifies a range:

- Breast cancer screening aims to detect disease at an early stage using radiological examination.
- Colorectal cancer has been screened for by providing the population with a list of

signs and symptoms that may alert them to changes that may indicate a cancer. A national screening programme for men and women over 60 years of age will detect blood in stools that may be caused by a cancer.

- Cervical cancer screening does not aim to detect the disease, but rather abnormalities that could lead to cancer.
- The Edinburgh Post-Natal Depression Scale assists primary care workers to identify those mothers who are suffering from depression.

We need to explore how decisions are made about which problems to screen for. Why screen for one disease and not another?

Why did screening develop?

When initially introduced into health care, screening only really extended the therapeutic range. This was obviously based on the idea that the outcome could potentially be improved if a disease process could be identified and treatment started at an early stage.

In diagrammatic terms this could be shown as:

A Without screening programme:	B With screening programme:
Pathological changes System presentation Diagnosis Treatment	Pathological changes Screening Diagnosis Treatment

Note the hoped-for difference in time from pathological changes occurring to treatment taking place between A and B.

Although screening continues to have the function of identifying pathological changes in at-risk individuals before symptoms present, it has also progressed to aim to prevent the onset of a disease altogether.

C   At risk of disease process
Screen
Prevent disease occurrence / action to reduce risk

An example of screening framework B would be cervical screening and an example of framework C would be genetic screening used in the preconceptual period. Try thinking of some more examples in Exercise 10.2.

There are several different types of screening format. Some types of screening need to be carried out in a specific time scale, i.e., phenylketonuria (a hereditary enzyme deficiency) screening must be carried out shortly after birth as severe mental

---

Exercise 10.2

Identify your own example of a screening programme that would fit into frame B and frame C:

B:
C:

---

deficiency would result if the diet was not amended immediately. Other screening tests are not restricted to specific time scales and in fact can be carried out opportunistically, i.e., whenever the opportunity presents. Some screening tests only need to be carried out once in a lifetime, others need to be repeated regularly. The whole population could potentially benefit from some screening programmes, others are targeted at a specific section of the population or one sex. Some examples of different screening formats are shown in Table 10.1:

Table 10.1 Examples of different screening formats

	Infant Hearing	Cervical	PKU	BSE	Questionnaire
ONCE ONLY			+		
REPEATED		+		+	
SELF				+	+
OPPORTUNISTIC				+	
UNIVERSAL	+		+		
SELECTIVE		+			
TIME SPECIFIC	+		+		

Notes: PKU = Phenylketonuria; BSE = breast self-examination.

We've explored a definition of screening and identified some of the forms it can take. The next question to address is, 'How are screening issues selected'? In other words, why do we only screen for some diseases and not all?

Exercise 10.3

Consider the following statement:

As long as sufficient finance is available, screening programmes should be established for every disease process.

Is it *true* or *false*?

The statement is in fact *false* because the development of a screening programme is not solely dependent on the availability of finance. Effective screening requires knowledge of the disease process as well as information on those at risk and the availability of effective treatment.

The UK National Screening Committee has the responsibility to draw on available evidence to identify programmes that 'do more good than harm'.

Screening criteria

Several criteria must be considered in any screening programme development. They may or may not all be met.

- there must be an identified need;
- the problem must present with sufficient frequency;
- it must be possible to identify those at risk;
- the test must be acceptable to the population at risk;
- the screening test must be reliable and valid;
- an acceptable and effective intervention must be available;
- the outcome for early intervention must be superior to that available when symptoms present naturally;
- the cost : benefit ratio must be acceptable.

We now need to explore some of the many issues involved in this list of screening criteria.

There must be an identified need

Usually, although not necessarily, this will be a disease process threatening individual and/or public health. For example, mass X-ray screening programmes were introduced in the 1940s when tuberculosis was a major threat to individual and public health, but were withdrawn in the 1980s when the threat of the disease had diminished.

Prostate cancer is recognized as an important health problem and it would be useful to be able to screen the population for the disease, but at present the UK National Health Service (NHS) does not consider that other screening criteria are met. For this reason screening is confined to a risk management strategy where men who are concerned about the disease can access the PSA Informed Choice Programme (see Further reading).

Exercise 10.4

Is there an established screening programme for prostate cancer in your country?

There is an acceptable screening test

The test itself must have certain qualities, such as being easy to perform, which could reduce the possibility of tester error, an acceptable financial cost, and an acceptable experience for the individuals being screened. For example, consider the options in Exercise 10.5.

Exercise 10.5

Consider how likely you would be to participate in a screening programme that involved:

- providing a urine sample once per year at a local venue;
- undergoing an examination under general anaesthetic once per year.

Presumably the level of personal discomfort and inconvenience would be important factors. However, these considerations would no doubt be tempered by your perceived level of risk of actually suffering from a particular disease. We'll develop these issues further later in the chapter.

Many difficult decisions may be encountered in relation to establishing screening programmes. Debates about the provision of screening programmes have ethical, moral, political and economic dimensions. Considerable emotions can be aroused when a screening test is in the process of being evaluated prior to full implementation. If the screening test proves to meet all the screening programme criteria, then some lives may have been lost because it has not been made generally available. On the other hand too early an implementation could generate a great deal of anxiety and inappropriate health care interventions. An example of this is the case of national mammography screening for breast cancer. In 1978, the Department of Health and Social Services in the UK set up randomized control trials to try to establish the most effective method of breast cancer screening, however, these trials were not complete when the group advising the government on the establishment of national breast screening (Forrest Report) was set up. Several other trials were also continuing in other parts of the world. However, it has been said that public and political pressure, the strong voicing of the fear that lives could be being lost while waiting for more evidence of the benefits of national mammography screening, led to implementation of the programme despite the existence of some medical doubts and uncertainties. The programme subsequently proved to be very effective.

There are international variations in operationalizing available screening tests. Comparison of the government recommendations relating to prostrate cancer is an interesting example (Table 10.2).

Table 10.2 International comparison of prostate cancer screening

Country	Recommendation
United Kingdom	Explicit policy not to offer this test
USA	Recommended every year for men >50 years
Canada	No recommendations
Australia	Not recommended

Source: Adapted from Jepson et al. (2000: 2).

An intervention strategy must be available

It would be totally unethical to develop and implement a screening test in order to identify a health problem for which there is no effective treatment strategy on offer.

The outcome for the disease is poor without early intervention

If there is an easy, cost-effective and successful treatment available for a disease it might be difficult to justify the professional, financial and personal investment involved in early identification through screening. It sounds straightforward common sense to say that screening should be used with those diseases having an improved out-come or prognosis as a consequence of early treatment. However, actually determining the benefits of early treatment is not as simple as it seems.

An important issue to clarify is, what exactly we mean by improved outcome, e.g. all of the following might be seen as improved outcome:

- more people are cured of a particular disease;
- survival time is increased;
- extension of the length of time that someone knows they are suffering from an illness without an actual improvement in survival time.

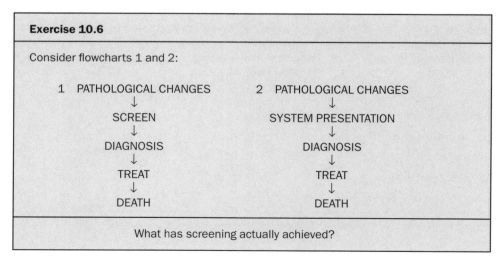

Exercise 10.6

Consider flowcharts 1 and 2:

1 PATHOLOGICAL CHANGES	2 PATHOLOGICAL CHANGES
↓	↓
SCREEN	SYSTEM PRESENTATION
↓	↓
DIAGNOSIS	DIAGNOSIS
↓	↓
TREAT	TREAT
↓	↓
DEATH	DEATH

What has screening actually achieved?

What we are actually talking about here is 'lead time', which refers to the situation in which survival time *appears* to have improved simply because screening has led to the disease being diagnosed earlier that it would have presented symptoms. You can see that assumptions about the effectiveness of screening can be complicated by using survival from time of diagnosis as a baseline measurement. This is not the only complicating factor when trying to determine the benefit of early diagnosis and treatment. For example, it may be that screening which takes place at three- to four-yearly intervals picks up a less aggressive form of a disease, e.g., cancer. Thus again screening may *appear* to increase survival simply because screening is picking up less aggressive diseases. We also need to give some thought to the individuals who present for screening, if the group who present have a higher incidence of the disease, i.e. if the rates of cervical cancer and breast cancer are different in different social classes, then the identification and treatment rate would also be affected.

Targeting a screening programme

In view of the issues we've just discussed, it is clear that targeting of a screening programme is an important issue. Randomized controlled trials provide some information on the effectiveness of tests with different individuals, timescales for screening, etc.

We can use the example of mammography screening for breast cancer to demonstrate this. There is currently some debate about what age group of women to invite for screening and how often screening should take place. Comparison of the outcome of screening for different age groups indicates screening appears to reduce mortality from breast cancer for women aged 50–69 but the advantages to younger women are less clear.

Prevalence by geographical location is another factor that can be used to target screening programmes. This is the case with sickle cell and thalassaemia screening in the UK where prevalence rates vary significantly across the country, as shown in Table 10.3.

Table 10.3 Estimates of % prevalence per annum by the Strategic Health Authority

Strategic Health Authority (SHA)	Pregnant women carrying significant haemoglobin variants (%)	Total no. of conceptions with sickle cell disorders
South-east London	6	51
North central London	6	30
Birmingham	3	11
Greater Manchester	2	6
Cumbria and Lancashire	<1	<1

Source: Adapted from NHS Sickle Cell & Thalassaemia Screening Programme, 2004.

High prevalence areas will offer routine screening, low prevalence SHAs will only screen based on an assessment of risk.

The screening test itself must have certain qualities

Screening tests must be reliable, in other words if the test is repeated on the same person the results should be consistent. The test must also be valid. Two measures of validity are sensitivity and specificity:

- test *sensitivity* is its ability to test true positives, i.e., to identify disease that is actually present;
- test *specificity* is its ability to identify true negatives, i.e., when the test result says the disease is not present, it definitely is not present.

A screening test may have both high specificity and high sensitivity, the ideal situation. However, this is not always the case. Consider them further in Exercise 10.7.

Exercise 10.7

Sensitivity and specificity determine how many true or false positives/negative can be expected from a test.

What would be the situation with a test with high sensitivity but low specificity?

What about a test with high specificity and low sensitivity?

Which of the above two tests is preferable for screening?

A test with high sensitivity but low specificity would identify most of the people in a population with the disease, but would be less useful at identifying those without the disease. In other words there would be a large number of false positives, people who were positive on the test but did not actually have the disease. In a test with high specificity but low sensitivity, the situation is reversed. The test is good at identifying those without the disease but less helpful at identifying those with the disease, i.e., there will be many false negatives – people negative on the test who do in fact have the disease. The ideal situation of course is to have a test which is highly sensitive and specific, but life is rarely like this. So if the choice is between high sensitivity and low specificity and high specificity and low sensitivity, which is the best test? The answer is that it depends on the consequence of making the wrong decision. If the condition is worth screening for, then picking up all (or as near to all as possible) people who may have the disease, with those who don't being excluded by further tests, would seem the best option. However, a screening strategy based on a sensitive but not very specific test could become prohibitively expensive. Expensive in the sense of health care resources devoted to excluding the false positives. But also expensive to the false positives in terms of unnecessary worry that they may have a serious disease, and time, discomfort and possibly serious risk of further medical investigation.

There must be a strong likelihood that those at risk will participate in the screening offered

Even if a particular screening test is responding to a significant need, has acceptable levels of sensitivity and specificity, etc., unless it can be feasibly expected that those people at risk can be identified, contacted and will actually participate in screening, the programme would not be worthwhile or effective.

If the population at risk is in routine contact with the screener, then the screening has the potential for greater impact and efficiency. For example, all babies born in the UK are screened for phenylketonuria, sickle cell disorders, thalassaemia and congenital hypothyroidism in hospital or by the community midwife; the screening programme has a virtually captive audience. Another example of a screening that can achieve high levels of participation is screening for postnatal depression offered to all women at six to eight weeks postpartum using the Edinburgh Postnatal Depression Score. These women are routinely in contact with primary care services and the screening tool is a questionnaire and not a physically invasive procedure that may create some discomfort. Comparison of this type of screening with a type that requires individuals to be individually selected and contacted to invite participation and the potential efficiency problems becomes apparent. Consider four scenarios in Exercise 10.8.

Compare your responses in Exercise 10.8 with the following suggestions (these responses are by no means complete, but raise some of the issues involved):

Example 1 criteria

- Significant number of at-risk individuals and public health risk.
- Migrants are an easily identifiable population.
- There is a valid test available to screen for the disease.
- The test is probably acceptable to those requiring screening.
- There is an effective treatment available for the disease.

Example 2 criteria

- It may be difficult to identify the target population.
- Selection of conditions to screen for would be available.
- We have no details yet from reading the content of the screening test and it would therefore be difficult to make a judgement as to its acceptability.
- Are we to assume that the possible intervention is termination of pregnancy or is there some other form of intervention, and exactly what would this involve in personal and economic terms?
- In order to say if the outcome from early intervention is superior, we would have to become involved in value, ethical, religious judgements, e.g., in relation to learning disabilities.

More information is really required before any decisions about screening programmes could be made.

Exercise 10.8

Four examples of issues for which it may be appropriate to develop screening pro-grammes are discussed below. Identify which screening criteria are present, and which would not be met and any other information required to make a decision about screening for the particular problem.

Example 1
Tuberculosis continues to be a health problem, although treatment opportunities are generally good. Nearly half the notifications for the disease in England and Wales are migrants from countries with high incidence of TB. Consequently migrants are forced to participate in screening at port health control units and their destination area is also informed to allow follow-up by community health personnel, i.e., a health visitor.
Criteria:

Example 2
There have recently been considerable advances in gene location knowledge. It may consequently be possible to theoretically develop genetic screening programmes. However, assuming some prioritization has to occur, should the screening be provided for the most severe forms of genetic disease or the most commonly occurring? There are numerous programmes underway to develop treatment programmes for various genetic diseases. Identifying the population who would benefit from screening may be a problem, because until someone gives birth to a child with a genetic problem, they may not be aware that they are carriers.
Criteria:

Example 3
A primary health care team are concerned that the population they serve may be con-suming unhealthy levels of alcohol. They would like to identify those concerned to try to assist them to reduce their levels of alcohol consumption. They are considering opportunistic screening or mailing out a questionnaire.
Criteria:

Example 4
Some countries in Europe have started experimental screening for a certain type of cancer. This particular type of cancer has a poor prognosis with late diagnosis, although developments in treatment in recent years have shown some improvement. Economic constraints on research are often named as an inhibitor to further treatment develop-ment. If this screening programme is effective, it could have a major impact on mortality from this disease, however, results so far are not conclusive.
Criteria:

Example 3 criteria

- The team appear to have identified a need, although it only appears to be based on assumptions.
- The test they seem to have in mind is one of questioning individuals about their alcohol consumption either in person or by questionnaire. Some people may want to participate in this, others may not.
- It would be difficult to verify the accuracy of the responses received.
- The effectiveness of a health promotion strategy to address alcohol consumption is not certain.

Example 4 criteria

- The outcome of treatment is improved with early diagnosis and treatment.
- We are uncertain as to whether the screening test is reliable or valid. There is obviously an ethical dilemma that if the screening turns out to be successful and we have not implemented it until after the experimental period, many lost lives could have been saved.

One of the screening criteria we have identified is that of the test being acceptable to those at risk. Another major factor to consider in any discussion on screening is participation. It doesn't necessarily follow that at risk groups will participate in a screening programme available to them.

Why do individuals participate in screening?

Start to answer the question by asking yourself why you have or why you would ever consider participating in screening.

People may participate in screening to be reassured that they are healthy, or to discover that they have a health problem. The former motive is probably the stronger. In order to deliberately expose yourself to the knowledge that your health is under threat you must:

- be aware of your risk;
- consider the risk to be sufficiently great;
- have confidence that there is an acceptable treatment available to you;
- believe the screening procedure has to be sufficiently accessible and acceptable.

Experience and research have identified several factors that appear to influence participation in screening. Gender seems to be an important factor in that men seem more reluctant than women to attend, but it's also more likely that women will have more contact with health care professionals perhaps because of family planning or child care needs. Attenders and non-attenders seem to hold different beliefs about control and fatalism in respect to health. Other apparently significant factors include: level of education, age, marital status and number of dependants. A systematic review of the determinants of screening uptake and interventions for increasing uptake contributes to the evidence base for practice (Jepson et al. 2000). Once someone has attended a screening, they are likely to do so again. Concentration on facilitating first attendance might therefore be sensible. Communication strategies such as supplementing letters with phone calls could be considered. This could be extended beyond pure reminders to the level of telephone counselling about factors inhibiting screening participation. Addressing any cost barriers to participation might also impact on screening uptake. A review of the cervical screening programme in Britain raises a number of these issues. Britain introduced a cervical screening programme in the 1960s. In 1988, the Department of Health instructed health authorities to establish computerized call–recall systems to try to ensure that those most at risk were invited to attend for screening. Providing someone with an automatic reminder could facilitate making the healthy choice the easy choice. However, if a woman has concerns or fears about attending, then receiving repeated reminders without any other supporting or informative communication could be seen to be anxiety-provoking.

This discussion on participation must also include questions on informed choice and freedom of participation. The systematic review produced by Jepson et al. (2000) identified limited evidence on client knowledge development as an outcome or as a determinant to uptake. Actual participation is often the criteria by which a screening service is evaluated. Few targets or evaluation measures address informed participation decision-making. This leads us to ask: 'Is or should participation in screening be through free choice?' Should it always be up to the individual to decide whether to participate or should any level of pressure be exerted on them? If it is more cost effective for society in general to treat a disease at an early stage, i.e., in terms of health care costs, sick leave costs, etc., should individuals be allowed free choice in participation? Consider this in Exercise 10.9.

Exercise 10.9

Consider the following examples and make a judgement as to the level of free choice that should be available. There are no right or wrong answers, this is an opportunity for you to consider some of the emotions, ethics and complexities involved.

How much choice should parents be given in participating in developmental screening for their children or hearing screening for their infants?

What level of persuasion should be used for women to attend for cervical screening? What happens in your area when women fail to attend? Are they offered a repeat invitation, does a health visitor make a home visit? Does the GP attempt to persuade the individual the next time they attend the surgery, even when they attend for an unrelated issue?

What is assumed to be the most responsible action from a pregnant woman who is at high risk of passing a genetic disease to her child, assuming there is screening available for that particular disease?

Is it reasonable to expect a 39-year-old mother expecting her first child to undertake amniocentesis screening, especially as the only 'cure' to a positive result is termination of pregnancy?

Summary

Working through the chapter should have helped you to answer the questions posed at the beginning. You can use the following headings to summarize the most important aspects of the chapter for you.

1   Give a definition of screening.

2   What are the principles guiding decisions about why we screen for some diseases and not others?

3   Drawing on your knowledge of why people do or don't participate in screening, list four reasons why a screening programme may have a high participation rate:

   •

   •

   •

   •

4   List four reasons why a screening programme may have a low participation rate:

   •

   •

   •

   •

You may wish to investigate these issues further and if so, you could collect information about the uptake rates of national or local screening programmes and suggest some explanations for the rates.

5   Complete the table below, using the example already provided earlier in the chapter to guide you:

	HIV	Amniocentesis	TB	Parenting problems	75+
Once only					
Repeated					
Self					
Opportunistic					
Universal					
Selective					
Time specific					

Now reflect again on what your skills and knowledge currently are, where there are gaps and any actions arising.

Public health standards	
Surveillance & assessment	
Promoting & protecting	
Developing quality & risk management	
Collaborative working for health	
Developing programmes & services & reducing inequalities	
Policy & strategy development & implementation	
Working with & for communities	
Strategic leadership	
Research & Development	
Ethically managing self, people & resources	

11

Changing public health: what impacts on public health practice?

How is evidence used to set priorities and to change public health practice?

How does perception of risk influence priority setting in public health?

How do various stakeholders influence the process of priority setting and public health practice?

How can the impact of public health practice be measured?

After working through this chapter you should be able to:

- provide an idealized account of how evidence is used to inform public health practice;
- provide examples of how in real life evidence is often not, or is incompletely, translated into public health practice;
- discuss other influences on the translation of evidence into public health practice, including the perception of risk and the interests of different stakeholders;
- discuss the importance of, and approaches to, evaluating the impact of public health practice in order to inform practice in the future;
- identify core skills required by public health professionals.

Introduction

This chapter aims to bring together many threads from previous chapters to consider how evidence, such as disease burden, disease determinants and the effectiveness of interventions, impacts on public health practice. Earlier, public health was defined as 'the art and science of preventing disease, promoting health and prolonging life through organized efforts of society'. Public health therefore covers a very broad range of interventions, for example, from the organized delivery of health care through to legislative or fiscal measures aimed at modifying patterns of unhealthy consumption, such as the smoking of tobacco.

The processes through which evidence is translated into public health practice are complex and in general remain poorly understood. They are as much about the art of public health as the science. In this chapter we hope to give some insight into how evidence impacts upon priority settings and changes in public health practice. We hope that this will enable you to reflect on, and look further into, approaches that you can use in your own work.

An idealized description of how evidence changes public health practice is illustrated in Figure 11.1. This description has five major stages:

1   Assessing the nature, severity and distribution of poor health states and their determinants within the population or group of interest.

2   Assessing which poor health states are amenable to improvement based on current knowledge and which are not.

3   The identification or development of interventions to tackle the poor heath states and, based on available resources, choosing the best mix of interventions that will achieve the maximum improvement in health.

4   Implementation of the interventions.

5   Monitoring the success of implementing the interventions and their impact upon population health, leading back to the start of the cycle.

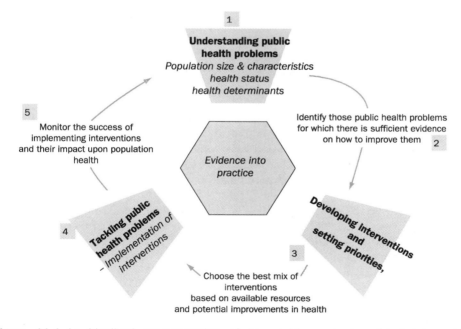

Figure 11.1 An idealized representation of how evidence is translated into public health practice

Note: Stages 1 to 5 are described in the text.

The process outlined in Figure 11.1 assumes a highly rationale approach to the translation of evidence into public health practice. In reality, of course, the process is much more complex. Below we consider the influences of risk perception and of competing interests of different stakeholders on the setting of public health priorities and the implementation of interventions.

Risk perception and priority setting

The perceived size of a threat is one very important element that affects human behaviour. Risk assessment plays a key role in priority setting. Risk assessment has been discussed in other sections of the book. Risk can be defined simply as the probability of an event occurring. However, perceived risk from a particular threat and the actual probability of that threat occurring often bear little relation to each other. Look now at Exercise 11.1.

Exercise 11.1

Think about the risk of death due to the following and put them into risk order starting with the lowest:

- Homicide
- Cancer
- Pregnancy
- Flood
- Tornado
- Road traffic accidents
- Heart disease
- Smallpox vaccination

Typically, you are likely to over-estimate the risk from unusual or dramatic events (e.g., floods; tornados; rare and particularly infectious diseases) and under-estimate the risk from common killers, such as heart disease. The order should have been: heart disease, cancer, road traffic accidents, homicide, pregnancy, flood, tornado, smallpox vaccination.

Why, then, do most people wrongly assess risk? The answer to this question is not straightforward and will differ between individuals. A range of factors has been associated with 'risk amplification', the perception of a risk being greater than it is. Figure 11.2 illustrates two interrelated factors in risk amplification: the extent to which the exposure to risk is voluntary, impersonal or imposed; and the degree of control that one perceives as having over the risk. Some people, for example, have a fear of flying and prefer to travel by road, even over long distances. They may perceive themselves as having much greater control over the risk associated with road travel even though in reality the risk associated with air travel is many times lower.

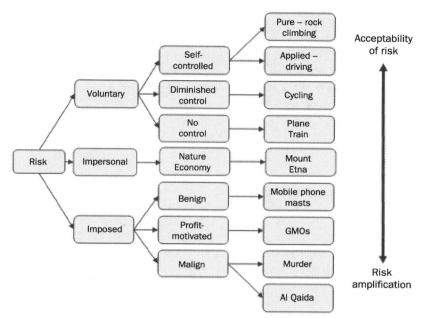

Figure 11.2 Illustration of factors involved in risk acceptability and risk amplification

Source: Taken from John Adams (2005).

Peter Bennett and Kenneth Calman in their book, *Risk Communication and Public Health*, list the following fright factors that are generally associated with people being more worried:

1 Involuntary exposure to a risk (i.e., pollution).
2 Risk is inequitably distributed (some benefit, others suffer).
3 Inescapable risk, no preventative precaution.
4 Risk from unfamiliar, novel sources.
5 Risk from sources that are man-made as opposed to natural.
6 Risk that affects women and small children.
7 A death perceived as being particularly dreadful.
8 Risk that affects identifiable as opposed to anonymous victims.
9 Risks that are poorly understood by science.
10 Risks that are presented by contradictory statements from responsible sources.

Reflect on how risk perception may influence public health decision-making, or the success of public health interventions by looking at Exercise 11.2.

Exercise 11.2

Can you think of any examples, such as from your own professional experience or national policy-making, where it appears that risk amplification has either driven public health decision-making or influenced the uptake of public health measures?

There are many examples you may have thought of in Exercise 11.2. In Britain, during the scare over mad cow disease[1] the government banned the sale of beef on the bone. This was on the grounds that the infective agent may be present in the bone, even though it was widely acknowledged that the risk of death in reality was very small, much less than a great number of other everyday activities that remained within the law. On reflection, it is clear the risks regarding mad cow disease were communicated to the public in a way which tended to amplify them greatly, with the media playing a large role in fuelling public concern. The banning of beef on the bone was at least in part the reaction of a government that wanted to be seen to be doing something.

An example of how risk perception may influence the uptake of public health measures is the refusal of some parents to have their children immunized against some infectious diseases. Both of these examples also raise other important issues, in particular on the roles of individual responsibility and free choice. In objecting to the ban on beef on the bone many people argued that they should be allowed to choose to eat beef on the bone if they wished, because for them the risk was acceptably low. Some people, controversially, will describe parents who refuse to have their children immunized as irresponsible on two grounds: first, on the grounds that the risk to their child from the disease is much greater than from the immunization; and second, with the argument that if large numbers of children are not immunized, then population-wide protection (often called 'herd immunity') breaks down and epidemics of that disease become possible again.

The politics of public health decision-making

Medicine is a social science and politics is nothing but medicine writ large!

This widely quoted statement was made by the famous German pathologist Virchow over 150 years ago. He was making the point that if medicine (in modern terms we would more appropriately use 'public health') is to be successful, then it must enter political and social life. He recognized, as discussed in Chapter 7, that the underlying determinants of health lie within the political, economic and social make-up of society. Therefore it should not be a surprise that public health decision-making, and

---

[1] A degenerative brain disease known as bovine spongiform encephalopathy, the infective agent of which is linked in humans to the degenerative brain disease called variant Creutzfeldt-Jacob disease (CJD).

the implementation of public health measures, are rarely as straightforward as the rational approach outlined in Figure 11.1 suggests. Look now at Box 11.1.

Box 11.1 Public health evidence and public health practice: the example of asbestos

The first published evidence linking occupational exposure to asbestos and lung disease appeared in the *British Medical Journal* in 1924: William Cook wrote of the illness and death of Nellie Kershaw who had worked in the spinning room of an asbestos factory. In 2000, Brazil, China, India, Japan, Russia and Thailand were consuming more than 60,000 tonnes of asbestos per year, accounting for more than 80 percent of the world's consumption. Many scientists have called for an international ban on the use of asbestos, but only a small number of countries have so far banned asbestos outright: Sweden, Norway, France, Germany, Poland and Saudi Arabia. It is predicted that the number of deaths from mesothelioma among men in Western Europe will increase from 7000 in 1998 to about 9000 by the year 2018, leading to a total of 250,000 by 2035.

So why has the evidence linking asbestos exposure with lung cancer and mesothelioma not been fully used to inform policy so many decades after it was proven? Who are the stakeholders that have influenced the debate and policy decisions for this preventable epidemic of illness and death?

Asbestos mining started in 1872 after it was discovered that a 10 percent addition of asbestos fibres to cement (asbestos cement) improved durability. During the twentieth century asbestos was an integral part of the industrialization process with global production peaking in 1975 at five million metric tons. Its uses were plentiful: insulation, drinking water pipes, brake lining, fireproofing, roofing material, heat insulation, etc. The asbestos industry has for many years argued that: (a) alternatives to asbestos were not available; (b) the majority of workers were smokers and therefore had inflicted a large part of their risk themselves; and (c) careful risk management was a cost-effective alternative.

The International Labour Organisation (ILO), a UN body, has been an important stakeholder by issuing Convention No. 162 concerning the safety of asbestos. The Scandinavian countries and the UK created national compulsory registers for mesothelioma deaths which allowed them to map asbestos imports against disease occurrence, documenting clearly how the epidemic mirrors the rise and fall of asbestos imports.

Consumers in developed countries are likely to continue to demand asbestos-based products because of their low cost and durability. From a public health point of view, it is desirable that they are given appropriate information about asbestos and its alternatives, reducing demand and consequently the mining and production of asbestos.

The description in Box 11.1 illustrates that although the dangers of asbestos have been known for over 80 years, and several countries have banned its use completely, it continues to be widely used in many countries. Several 'stakeholders' have strongly supported its continued use, including not surprisingly asbestos mining companies, the manufacturers of asbestos-based products and consumers who use those products. There also appears to be the sense in some countries that the risk associated with the use of asbestos is acceptable when put alongside some of the advantages of asbestos-based products (even though alternatives exist).

The example in Box 11.1 illustrates that decisions affecting the public are highly influenced by the interests (often competing interests) of groups vs. individuals within society. The term 'stakeholder' is often used to describe such groups or individuals. The term 'stakeholder' is used here to refer to any person, group or institution that can influence or be influenced by a public health measure. Their influence may work in favour of public health or against it. Sometimes the activities of stakeholders can be underhand, deliberately pursuing their own interests at the expense of public health. In recent history, the activities of the tobacco industry provide the clearest example of this. For example, it is well documented that the industry attempted to deliberately mislead the public on the dangers of tobacco, and that it uses its huge commercial power in attempts to modify government policy – most recently in developing countries where it is seeking new markets to replace falling cigarettes sales in developed countries.

Figure 11.3 provides some examples of stakeholders relevant to public health. It is sometimes useful to categorize stakeholders as primary and secondary. A primary stakeholder is one who is directly affected by a public health programme or intervention, whether for good or for ill. A secondary stakeholder is one who has some role or influence, whether positive or negative, explicit or implicit, on the success of implementing a public health programme or intervention.

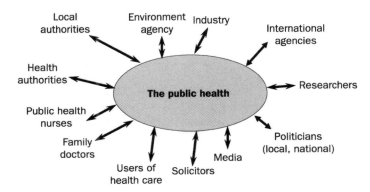

Figure 11.3 Examples of public health stakeholders

Undertaking a stakeholder analysis is usually an essential step in planning a public health intervention. Such an analysis enables one to plan strategically how to deal with different groups who can influence the success of the intervention. Such an analysis might identify for each stakeholder their key interests relevant to the intervention, the support and action (if any) that are desired from that stakeholder in order to ensure the success of the intervention and what is required to try ensure that stakeholders respond appropriately.

Exercise 11.3

For a particular public health issue of interest to you, complete a stakeholder analysis using the framework below. Show additional stakeholders as necessary

Stakeholder	Key interests of stakeholder relevant to the public health issue	Support and action desired from the stakeholder by you	Actions required by you
Environment agency			
Local authority			
Health authority			
Family doctors			
Public health nurses			
Industry			
International agencies			
Researchers			
Politicians			
Media			
Solicitors			
Service users			

Use Exercise 11.3 to think about a public health issue that is of interest or concern to you and undertake a stakeholder analysis using the framework given. Clearly, depending on the issue, not all the potential stakeholders listed in the table may be involved, and there may be other stakeholders to add who are not listed there.

Evidence and public health practice

This chapter began by considering an idealized, technical model on how evidence impacts upon public health practice. However, we have seen that public health practice is influenced by much more than the type of evidence considered in that model.

Perceptions of risk and the competing interests of different stakeholders are two areas that have a great impact on decisions affecting the public health.

In the last section of this chapter we consider approaches to determining whether public health measures actually have the impact that was intended.

Assessing if we are addressing the right public health needs in the right way

How can we assess if we are meeting priorities and that any public health action is having the desired impact? One way is to ensure that we use a range of evidence to inform practice. Figure 11.4 provides a summary of some of the main types of evidence that are relevant and useful to public health practice.

	Understanding public health problems		Setting priorities and develop interventions					
Evidence on health states and health gain	Descriptive and aetiological epidemiology	Qualitative studies of health and behaviours	Qualitative studies of interventions	Efficacy and effectiveness studies, including cost effectiveness	*Economic evaluation*	*Implementation research*	*Policy evaluation*	*Quality of life research*
Evidence on public involvement	Risk assessment; risk perception; risk communication	Stakeholder analyses Patient preferences	Public and other stakeholder preferences for different options Decision analysis in clinical care					

Figure 11.4 Summary of some of the main types of evidence relevant to public health practice (based on a model developed by M. White)*

Note: * With thanks to Professor Martin White, School of Population and Health Sciences, Newcastle University.

Notice that in the so-called idealized and technical model shown in Figure 11.1, the type of evidence considered largely concerned the size of public health problems and evidence on the effectiveness of interventions to address them. However, as discussed above, such evidence provides only part of what is required to inform public health practice. For example, knowledge on the perception of risk, and on the interests, activities and preferences of major stakeholders is also needed to plan public health interventions. This type of evidence is flagged in Figure 11.4 under the heading of 'evidence on public involvement'. It includes studies of risk perception, analyses of the roles and interests of stakeholders, and studies on the preferences of stakeholders, including patients and health carers, for different options. Look now at Exercise 11.4.

Exercise 11.4

Consider a public health issue that you are familiar with, and use the boxes in Figure 11.4 to think through all the evidence that is currently available for it and list this below.

Identify areas where evidence is lacking.

Had you previously considered all of these areas?

If not, does your understanding change at all when you take them into account?

Measuring the impact of public health action can be a complex and challenging task. Let us start with a straightforward example such as immunizations against infectious diseases. It is possible to identify a population at risk, provide the vaccine and measure the incidence of the disease. A safe vaccine and a reduction in the disease would be good indicators of a positive and successful impact having been made.

Let us consider another example: breast cancer screening. We would not expect this public health intervention to have any impact on incidence of the disease, but rather on the mortality rate. A reduction in mortality rates from breast cancer in a population where screening is available can be partly attributed to the screening process. However, a reduction may also be attributable to increased provision of cancer specialists and so rapid treatment; it may also be attributed to improved lifestyle habits, such as in diet, which may impact on the likelihood of developing cancer; it may be attributable to raised awareness in the population not offered screening but who undertake self-examination.

There is a considerable evidence base on effective ways to tackle public health needs. For example, in the United Kingdom the National Institute for Health and Clinical Excellence (NICE) provides details on a range of public health evidence. One of the challenges faced by public health practitioners is that the expected impact of an intervention now may not be fully apparent for maybe 20 or 30 years. A good example would be a balanced diet and adequate levels of exercise in childhood should lead to a reduction in coronary heart disease when the child is in their mid-life years. In some ways we can measure the potential of achieving this outcome during that time period, for example, by monitoring blood cholesterol levels and blood pressure levels. However, there is considerable room for the development of intermediate short-term impact measures, especially measures and approaches that are suitable for small-scale community development or area-based approaches to addressing public health needs. We'll explore this issue in the next section.

Developing evidence on effectiveness of interventions from public health practice

This section relates specifically to small-scale public health intervention. Capturing evidence from such projects is difficult, but it is possible and this provides a useful contribution to the evidence base. We want to consider two issues in particular, the effectiveness of individual interventions and the effectiveness of multiple interventions.

First, let us consider individual interventions. By this we mean activities such as running a walking group, a support group, a community kitchen. Projects such as these can only reasonably make a contribution to impacting on an aspect of a health determinant. An essential part of this type of public health practice is to identify a time line and a series of incremental health outcome achievements that would lead to the desired health outcome. The specific contribution that any individual intervention can make can then be clarified. In order to begin to reveal evidence of effectiveness, we have to use tools specific to the purpose. Such a tool could be the context–mechanism–outcome model (Pawson and Tilley 2004). Context refers to the particular situation in which the intervention will take place, the characteristics, needs, cultures and history. The mechanism is the specific intervention and delivery mode. Outcome is the result that occurs which would indicate that success had been achieved. The case study presented in Box 11.2 (facing) demonstrates how this could be used.

Let us move on to consider issues about measuring the effectiveness of multiple interventions. Evidence from this aspect of public health is generally not well addressed, partly because of lack of inter-agency planning and service provision. At any one time, in any one community, there are likely to be several public health interventions in action. Some will be targeting individual health, others population health issues. Reference to the work on complex community initiatives (Connell et al. 1995) highlights the need to acknowledge the potential for interaction between public health interventions and a synergy among them. However, many public health initiatives are established and evaluated individually, with insufficient acknowledgement of the contribution of other previous or concurrent interventions. Cumulative impact is therefore not well addressed. Tools such as health impact assessment which requires a consideration of the context in which any intervention is to take place enhances the opportunity for multiple impact and impact interaction recognition.

Skills for changing public health

To conclude this chapter it is useful to revisit areas of specialist public health practice and consider how they impact on developing evidence of public health need, determining priorities for public health action, developing and implementing interventions to respond to public health needs and the influencing of the whole process.

Areas of specialist public health practice

1   Surveillance and assessment of the population's health and well-being (including managing, analysing and interpreting information, knowledge and statistics).

Box 11.2 Case study demonstrating the context–mechanism–outcome model

An individual community development worker is charged with developing a public health intervention that will impact on the high levels of coronary heart disease in the locality. The project typically has only a small amount of funding and is time limited. It is important therefore to consider how to capture the impact this small-scale intervention achieves. Using epidemiological evidence of coronary heart disease rates would not be helpful. One reason is that there would be a considerable time delay in any change being manifested in rates. What would be useful would be to consider if an aspect of a lifestyle health determinant influencing coronary heart disease could be challenged. The worker would have to consider four questions:

1 *What evidence is there to identify which determinant to focus on?*
   What do we know about factors such as dietary habits in the area, what do we know about levels of exercise in the area? Which aspect of coronary heart disease health would it be wise to focus on? We'll assume that poor dietary habits are evident – there could be evidence from a health and lifestyle survey or it may be qualitative evidence from a health needs analysis.
2 *Which activities/interventions are likely to be effective and acceptable in this area?*
   Would a group approach to the intervention be sensible – are there any naturally occurring groups? What seems to be potentially having an influence on diet choice – access to shops, income to buy a 'healthy diet', are loneliness and isolation impacting on poor diet due lack of self-interest? If we assume that all these factors are present, the option of developing a community kitchen would seem a potentially acceptable intervention.
3 *What outcomes would indicate that the intervention had been effective?*
   A number of outcomes could indicate success. Reduction in isolation could be demonstrated in regular attendance at the community kitchen. An increase in the number of people choosing the food option cooked in the healthiest way such as grilled rather than fried based on an enhanced understanding of a healthy diet.
4 *Were these outcomes achieved and if not, why not?*
   Consideration of this question allows learning on what works in particular contexts and helps to enhance understanding of public health needs. The next step in the process would be to consider issues of sustainability and to clarify priorities for other interventions that would complement what had been achieved.

2 Promoting and protecting the population's health and well-being.
3 Developing quality and risk management within an evaluative culture.
4 Developing health programmes and services and reducing inequalities.
5 Working with and for communities.
6 Research and development.
7 Ethically managing self, people and resources (including education and continuing professional development).

8   Strategic leadership for health.

9   Policy and strategy development and implementation.

10   Collaborative working for health.

Exercise 11.5

Examples of how utilization of various public health skills can change public health are given below. There is also a blank column for you to identify your own examples that may be particularly relevant to you:

Skill	Example of utilization	Example of utilization
1	Combining evidence sources	
2	Developing specific outcomes for health promotion	
3	Developing mechanisms for communication of risk evidence to the public	
4	Integrating inequalities impact evaluation into service planning and delivery	
5	Contextualizing priority setting and intervention development	
6	Influencing the research agenda to ensure appropriate impact tools are developed	
7	Ensuring all stakeholder voices are heard	
8	Proactive and evidence-based approaches	
9	Cyclical evaluation activity	
10	Working with multiple stakeholders	

Summary

Working through this chapter should have helped you to answer the questions posed at the beginning. You can use the following headings to summarize the most important aspects of the chapter for you.

1   Select a public health issue relevant to your work and consider how evidence has been used to determine public health practice.

2   Using the same public health issue as in question 1, consider the range of stake-holders who have been influential in determining public health practice and how much their influence was based on public health evidence.

3   Select a public health issue that you regularly encounter in your area of work and review the evidence on this issue (you might use the NICE, see Further reading). Consider the challenges you face in using the available evidence to communicate with the relevant population. You need to include consideration of population perceptions of risk and how this may affect the process.

4   Using the four questions listed below, consider how you could apply the context–mechanism–outcome model to an aspect of your practice:

•   What evidence is there to identify which determinant to focus on?

•   Which activities/interventions are likely to be effective and acceptable in this area?

•   What outcomes would indicate that the intervention had been effective?

•   Were these outcomes achieved and if not, why not?

Further reading, references and resources

The epidemiological texts below are those that we think are particularly high quality, are clear and are consistent with the contents of the book. All the definitions used in the book, are consistent with those found in the *Dictionary of Epidemiology*, published by the International Epidemiological Association.

Chapter 1

Alfredo, M. (2004) *History of Epidemiologic Methods and Concepts*. Basel: Birkhäuser Verlag, 405 pages. (Combines a history of epidemiological methodology with a series of articles by contemporary epidemiologists on historical figures such as John Snow and William Farr.)

Beaglehole, R. and Bonita, R. (2004) *Public Health at the Crossroads: Achievements and Prospects*, 2nd edn. Cambridge: Cambridge University Press. (Very spirited account of global public health issues with good critiques of the interplay between public health and epidemiology.)

Buck, C., Llopis, A., Najera, E. and Terris, M. (eds) (1988) *The Challenges of Epidemiology: Issues and Selected Readings*, Scientific Publications No. 505. Washington, DC: Pan American Health Organization, 989 pages. (Very useful collation of almost 90 historical articles with commentaries.)

Committee of Inquiry into the Future Development of the Public Health Function (1988) *Public Health in England* (Acheson Report). London: HMSO, p. 289. (One of many reviews of the roles and responsibilities of public health within the tensions of the roles of states and individuals.)

Detels, R., McEwan, J., Beaglehole, R. and Tanaka, H. (eds) (2002) *Oxford Textbook of Public Health*, 4th edn. Oxford: Oxford University Press. (Standard text book with separate chapters for developed, developing and transition countries.)

Doll, R. and Hill, B. (2002) Smoking and carcinoma of the lung: a preliminary report, in *Oxford Textbook of Public Health*, 4th edn. Oxford: Oxford University Press, pp. 475–91.

Hamlin, C. (2002) The history and development of public health in developed countries, in *Oxford Textbook of Public Health*, 4th edn. Oxford: Oxford University Press, pp. 21–37.

International Network for the History of Public Health. Available at: http://www.liu.se/tema/inhph/ (Academic association of researchers in the field.)

Jenner, E. (2002) An inquiry into the causes and effects of variolae vaccinae, in *Oxford Textbook of Public Health*, 4th edn. Oxford: Oxford University Press, pp. 31–2.

Krieger, N. (1999) Questioning epidemiology: objectivity, advocacy, and socially responsible science, *American Journal of Public Health*, 89(8): 1151–3.

Kyoum Kim, D. and Yui, S.-Z. (2002) Countries in economic transition: a history and development of public health in China and Korea, in *Oxford Textbook of Public Health*, 4th edn. Oxford: Oxford University Press, pp. 63–80.

Last, J.M., Spasoff R.A. and Harris, S.S. (2000) *A Dictionary of Epidemiology*, 4th edn. London: International Epidemiology Association. (Classic resource for definitive definition of terms relating to epidemiology.)

Lind, J. (2002) An inquiry into the nature, causes and cure of the scurvy, in *Oxford Textbook of Public Health*, 4th edn. Oxford: Oxford University Press, pp. 20–3.

McKeown, T. (1976) *The Role of Medicine: Dream, Mirage or Nemesis?* London: The Nuffield Provincial Hospital Trust. (McKeown's observations are one of the classical texts that helped to explain the complex interplay of personal and societal risk factors for human disease.)

Porter, D. (1999) *Health, Civilisation and the State: A History of Public Health from the Ancient to the Modern*. London: Routledge, 376 pages. (Porter is a medical historian who has compiled a great deal of detail from a range of countries illuminating the early phases of public health thinking.)

Schwartz, S., Susser, E. and Susser, M. (1999) A future for epidemiology, *Rev. Public Health*, 20: 15–33.

Sein, T., and Rasei, U.M. (2002) The history and development of public health, in *Oxford Textbook of Public Health*, 4th edn. Oxford: Oxford University Press, pp. 39–61.

Snow, J. (1988) On the mode of communication of cholera, in Buck, C., Llopis, A., Najera, E. and Terris, M. (eds) *The Challenge of Epidemiology: Issues and Selected Readings*, Scientific Publications No. 505. Washington, DC: Pan American Health Organization.

Snow, John, website maintained by University College Los Angeles. Available at: http://www.ph.ucla.edu/epi/snow.html (Lots of very well-presented information useful at all levels.)

Susser, M. (1996) Choosing a future for epidemiology I: eras and paradigms, *American Journal of Public Health*, 86(5): 668–73.

Susser, M. (1998) Does risk factor epidemiology put epidemiology at risk? Peering into the future, *Journal of Epidemiology: Community Health*, 52: 608–11.

Vinten-Johansen, P., Brody, H., Paneth, N., Rashman, S. and Rip, M. (2003) *Cholora, Chloroform and the Science of Medicine: A Life of John Snow*. Oxford: Oxford University Press, 437 pages. (Very detailed and scholarly account of John Snow's life from his early years in the north of England to his later life in London.)

Chapter 2

Adult Morbidity and Mortality Project website: http://www.ncl.ac.uk/ammp/ (More details, including the major project reports, on the demographic surveillance system in Tanzania described in Box 2.1.)

Detels, R., Walter, W.H., McEwan, J. and Omenn, G.S. (eds) (1997) *Oxford Textbook of Public Health*, 3rd edn. Oxford: Oxford University Press. (See section 1 of volume 2 on information systems and sources of intelligence.)

Hansell, A., Bottle, A., Shurlock, L. and Aylin, P. (2001) Accessing and using hospital activity data, *Journal of Public Health Medicine*, 53: 51–6. (Useful article discussing the uses and limitations of hospital activity data within the UK. Many of the issues are relevant to similar data in other parts of the world.)

Health Protection Agency (England and Wales) website: http://www.hpa.org.uk/ (Details of the role of the Health Protection Agency, including communicable disease surveillance, and access to some of the data it collects and collates.)

Lippeveld, T., Sauerborn, R. and Bodart, C. (eds) (2000) *Design and Implementation of Health Information Systems*. Geneva: World Health Organisation.

Lwanga, S.K., Cho-Yook, T. and Ayeni, O. (1999) *Teaching Health Statistics: Lesson and Seminar Outlines*. Geneva: World Health Organisation. (Although designed as an aid to teaching about health statistics, it provides a very good overview of the major issues covered in this chapter, particularly the second part on 'Health statistics, including demography and vital statistics'.)

Office of National Statistics (UK) website: http://www.statistics.gov.uk/ (A very good source of data on a whole range of social, economic and health-related items. Includes links to resources describing the census procedures, registration of births and deaths, analyses of trends in deaths rates and causes of death, and so on.)

World Health Organisation Statistical Information System website: http://www3.who.int/whosis/ (This site provides access to a range of data provided by the World Health Organisation, including mortality and burden of disease data for all 192 member states. Also provides access to papers describing the methodology for some of the estimates, and to details of the international classification of diseases.)

World Health Organisation (2005) *Bulletin of the World Health Organization*, August, 83(8). Available at: http//www.who.int/bulletin/ (Special issue on health information systems, covering in particular approaches that meet the needs of low and middle income countries.)

Chapter 3

Bhopal, R.S. (2002) *Concepts of Epidemiology: An Integrated Introduction to the Ideas, Theories, Principles and Methods of Epidemiology*. Oxford: Oxford University Press. (A refreshing and clear approach to the principles and practice of epidemiology. Nicely illustrated with diagrammatic and pictorial examples.)

Hennekens, C.H. and Buring, J.E. (1987) *Epidemiology in Medicine*, S.L. Mayrent (ed.). Boston: Little and Brown. (Although published in 1987, this remains one of the clearest and most accessible accounts of major epidemiological concepts and study designs, including all the issues covered in this chapter.)

Last, J.M. Spasoff, R.A. et al. (2000) *A Dictionary of Epidemiology*, 4th edn. London: International Epidemiology Association.

Rothman, K. and Greenland, S. (1997) *Modern Epidemiology*, 2nd edn. Philadelphia: Lippincott-Raven. (Arguably the major reference text for epidemiology. Particularly strong on the theoretical underpinnings of study methodology and approaches to analysis.)

Supercourse – epidemiology, the internet and global health website: http://www.pitt.edu/~super1/ (This site provides a collection of over 2000 lectures, many from very good teachers of epidemiology, freely downloadable as PowerPoint presentations. They include lectures on areas covered in this chapter, such as measures of disease frequency and standardization of rates.)

Chapter 4

Bhopal, R.S. (2002) *Concepts of Epidemiology: An Integrated Introduction to the Ideas, Theories, Principles and Methods of Epidemiology*. Oxford: Oxford University Press. (A refreshing and clear approach to the principles and practice of epidemiology. Nicely illustrated with diagrammatic and pictorial examples.)

Hennekens, C.H. and Buring, J.E. (1987) *Epidemiology in Medicine*, S.L. Mayrent (ed.) Boston: Little and Brown. (Although published in 1987, this remains one of the clearest and most accessible accounts of major epidemiological concepts and study designs, including all the issues covered in this chapter.)

Last, J.M., Spasoff R.A. and Harris, S.S. (2000) *A Dictionary of Epidemiology*, 4th edn. London: International Epidemiology Association. (Classic resource for definitive definition of terms relating to epidemiology.)

Rothman, K. and Greenland, S. (1997) *Modern Epidemiology*, 2nd edn. Philadelphia: Lippincott-Raven. (Arguably the major reference text for epidemiology. Particularly strong on the theoretical underpinnings of study methodology and approaches to analysis.)

Supercourse – epidemiology, the Internet and global health website: http://www.pitt.edu/~super1/ (This site provides a collection of over 2000 lectures, many from very good teachers of epidemiology, freely downloadable as PowerPoint presentations. They include lectures on areas covered in this chapter, such as concepts and measures of risk.)

Chapter 5

Bhopal, R.S. (2002) *Concepts of Epidemiology: An Integrated Introduction to the Ideas, Theories, Principles and Methods of Epidemiology*. Oxford: Oxford University Press. (A refreshing and clear approach to the principles and practice of epidemiology. Nicely illustrated with diagrammatic and pictorial examples.)

Buck, C., Llopis, A., Najera, E. and Terris, M. (eds) (1988) *The Challenge of Epidemiology: Issues and Selected Readings*. Washington, DC: Pan American Health Organization (PAHO). (This book contains a collection of classic epidemiological papers, covering the range of study designs (and more) described in this chapter. A list of the contents of the book, with abstracts for each of the articles, can be found at: http://www.ingentaconnect.com/content/paho/chepi).

Hennekens, C.H. and Buring, J.E. (1987) *Epidemiology in Medicine*, S.L. Mayrent (ed.) Boston: Little and Brown. (Although published in 1987, this remains one of the clearest and most accessible accounts of major epidemiological concepts and study designs, including all the issues covered in this chapter.)

Last, J.M. Spasoff, R.A. et al. (2000) *A Dictionary of Epidemiology*, 4th edn. London: International Epidemiological Association.

Rothman, K. and Greenland, S. (1997) *Modern Epidemiology*, 2nd edn. Philadelphia: Lippincott-Raven. (Arguably the major reference text for epidemiology. Particularly strong on the theoretical underpinnings of study methodology and approaches to analysis.)

Supercourse – epidemiology, the internet and global health website: http://www.pitt.edu/~super1/ (This site provides a collection of over 2000 lectures, many from very good teachers of epidemiology, freely downloadable as PowerPoint presentations. They include lectures on areas covered in this chapter, and include lectures on each of the major types of epidemiological study design.)

Chapter 6

Bhopal, R.S. (2002) *Concepts of Epidemiology: An Integrated Introduction to the Ideas, Theories, Principles and Methods of Epidemiology*. Oxford: Oxford University Press. (A refreshing and clear approach to the principles and practice of epidemiology. Nicely illustrated with diagrammatic and pictorial examples.)

Hennekens, C.H. and Buring, J.E. (1987) *Epidemiology in Medicine*, S.L. Mayrent (ed.) Boston: Little and Brown. (Although published in 1987, this remains one of the clearest and most accessible accounts of major epidemiological concepts and study designs, including all the issues covered in this chapter.)

Last, J.M., Spasoff R.A. and Harris, S.S. (2000) *A Dictionary of Epidemiology*, 4th edn. London: International Epidemiology Association. (Classic resource for definitive definition of terms relating to epidemiology.)

Rothman, K. and Greenland, S. (1997) *Modern Epidemiology*, 2nd edn. Philadelphia: Lippincott-Raven. (Arguably the major reference text for epidemiology. Particularly strong on the theoretical underpinnings of study methodology and approaches to analysis.)

Supercourse – epidemiology, the internet and global health: website: http://www.pitt.edu/~super1/ (This site provides a collection of over 2000 lectures, many from very good teachers of epidemiology, freely downloadable as PowerPoint presentations. They include lectures on areas covered in this chapter, and include lectures on weighing up chance, bias and confounding and assessing causality.)

Chapter 7

Kuh, D., Ben-Shlomo, Y., Lynch, J., Hallqvist, J. and Power, C. (2003) Life course epidemiology, *Journal of Epidemiology and Community Health*, 57: 778–83. (A very useful introduction to some of the key concepts, written by people who have been instrumental in developing this field of study.)

Last, J.M., Spasoff R.A. and Harris, S.S. (2000) *A Dictionary of Epidemiology*, 4th edn. London: International Epidemiology Association. (Classic resource for definitive definition of terms relating to epidemiology.)

Mackenbach, J.P. (1994) The epidemiologic transition theory, *Journal of Epidemiology & Community Health*, 48: 329–31. (A critical review of the theory.)

Murray, C. and Lopez, A. (1996) *The Global Burden of Disease: A Comprehensive Assessment of Mortality and Disability from Diseases, Injuries, and Risk Factors in 1990 and Projected to 2020.* Geneva: World Health Organisation. (The original major publication describing the methodology for undertaking the study, including the derivation of DALY (Disability Adjusted Life Year). Several articles in the *Lancet* can also be found, and more information is available from the WHO statistics website (www3.who.int/.)

Olshansky, S.J. and Ault, A.B. (1986) The fourth stage of the epidemiologic transition: the age of delayed degenerative diseases, *Milbank Quarterly*, 64: 355–91. (The paper which suggested that a fourth stage should be added to the theory of the epidemiological transition.)

Omran, A.R. (1971) The epidemiologic transition: a theory of the epidemiology of population change, *Milbank Memorial Fund Quarterly*, 49: 509–38. (The original description of the theory of the epidemiological transition.)

Public Health Agency of Canada website (section on the determinants of population health): http://www.phac-aspc.gc.ca/ph-sp/phdd/determinants/ (An excellent web resource, covering the major determinants, with evidence for their role and examples of initiatives to address them.)

Supercourse – epidemiology, the internet and global health website: http://www.pitt.edu/~super1/ (This site provides a collection of over 2000 lectures, many from very good teachers of epidemiology, freely downloadable as PowerPoint presentations. Lectures relevant to this chapter include those on the epidemiological transition.)

United Nations (Human development reports) website: http://hdr.undp.org/reports/ (Access to data from the United Nations human development reports, some of it overlapping with the data available from the World Bank website.)

Wilkinson, R. and Marmot, M. (eds) (2003) *Social Determinants of Health*, 2nd edn. Geneva: World Health Organisation. Freely available as a PDF file from: http://www.who.dk/document/e81384.pdf (A comprehensive review of the social and economic determinants of health, largely written from the perspective of the situation in modern Western Europe and North America.)

World Bank Data and Statistics website: http://www.worldbank.org/data/ (Range of data by individual countries and groups of countries (e.g., by income category) on economic, social and health-related topics.)

World Health Organization (2001) *Macroeconomics and Health: Investing in Health for Economic Development. Report of the Commission on Macroeconomics and Health*. Geneva: World Health Organization. Available at: www.who.int (A search on 'Commission for Macroeconomics and Health' will pull up this and other relevant documents. This is a very influential report on the links between poverty and health, relevant in particular to differences in health between rich and poor countries. It includes discussion on the links between globalization and health.)

World Health Organization Statistical Information System website: http://www3.who.int/whosis/ (This site provides access to a range of data provided by the World Health Organization, including mortality and burden of disease data for all 192 member states, and broken down into low, middle and high income countries).

Chapter 8

Bauld, L. and Judge, K. (eds) (2002) *Learning from Health Action Zone*. Chichester: Aeneas. (This book is a collection of reports of experiences relating to the implication of HAZ. It addresses issues such as social capital, urban regeneration, and community development programmes.)

Beishon, M. (2005) Social marketing: brand new approach, *Health Development Today*, December/January. Available at: www.hda-online.org.uk/hdt

Carr, S. M. and Clarke, C. (2002) Guiding small-scale evaluation: a critical step in developing practice, *Practice Development in Health Care*, 1(2): 104–17. (The issues discussed in this paper generate from developing evaluation tools for a Health Action Zone. Many of the issues can be transferred to addressing evaluation of health promotion interventions.)

Dahlgren, G. and Whitehead, M. (1991) *Policies and Strategies to Promote Social Equity in Health*. Stockholm: Institute of Future Studies.

Department of Health (DoH) (2004) *Choosing Health: Making Healthy Choices Easier*. London: The Stationery Office (UK Government policy document.)

Health Development Agency website: www.hda.org.uk (Provides health promotion and public health news at regional and international levels and provides a number of related links.)

Health Development Agency Evidence Base website: www.hda-online.org.uk/evidence (This is a very useful resource for searching the evidence in relation to a health promotion need or intervention. It covers a wide range of issue such as 'Breast feeding for longer – what works?', 'Evidence of effective drug prevention in young people', 'The effectiveness of public health interventions for increasing physical activity'.)

Health Protection Agency website: www.hpa.org.uk (Provides information on agency activities and responsibilities, topical issues and has regional links.)

Scriven, A. and Garman, S. (eds) (2004) *Promoting Health: Global Perspectives*. London: Palgrave Macmillan. (Provides useful discussion of health issues at a global level and makes international comparisons of health challenges and approaches to health promotion.)

World Health Organisation website: www.who.org (Provides information on international health issues, targets and strategies. A useful exercise to trace the developing appreciation of health promotion on public health over time would be to access 'Declaration of Alma Ata 1978', ' Ottawa Charter 1986', 'Jakarta Declaration 1997'.)

World Health Organisation (2004) *Global Strategy on Diet, Physical Activity and Health*. Geneva: WHO. (This document considers the major non-communicable diseases challenging world health.)

Chapter 9

Bauld, L. and Judge, K. (eds) (2002) *Learning from Health Action Zone*. Chichester: Aeneas. (This book is a collection of reports of experiences relating to the implication of HAZ. It recounts experiences in relation to issues such as social capital, urban regeneration, engaging communities, community development programmes, and community involvement.)

Bradshaw, J. (1972) *The concept of social need*. New Society, 30 March.

Department of Health (1999) *Saving Lives: Our Healthier Nation*. London: Department of Health. (Provides a description on the state of the health of the population of England and Wales, identifies national priorities for action and sets targets.)

Department of Health (2001) *Shifting the Balance of Power within the NHS: Securing Delivery*. London: The Stationery Office. (Details Primary Care Trust responsibility to conduct HNA.)

Department of Health (2004) *Choosing Health: Making Healthy Choices Easier*. London: The Stationery Office.

Firkin, S.B., Lewando-Hundt, G. and Draper, A.K. (2000) *Participatory Approaches in Health Promotion and Health Planning: A Literature Review*. London: Health Development Agency. (Provides comprehensive details of the background, theory and applications of participatory approaches.)

Hamer, L. and Easton, N. (2002) *Community Strategies and Health Improvement: A Review of Policy and Practice*. London: Health Development Agency. (Provides discussion on policy context and examples of collaborative and partnership working.)

Health Development Agency website: www.hda-online.org.uk (The new National Institute for Health and Clinical Excellence (NICE) has taken on the functions of the Health Development Agency to create a single excellence-in-practice organization responsible for providing national guidance on the promotion of good health and the prevention and treatment of ill health.)

Health Development Agency (HDA) (2000) *Participatory Approaches in Health Promotion and Health Planning: Summary Bulletin*. London: HDA. (Provides basic introduction to participatory approaches, traces history and background and identifies key components of the process.)

Health Development Agency (HDA) (2002) *Introducing health impact assessment (HIA): informing the decision-making process*.

Health Development Agency (HDA) (2004a) *Social Capital*, HDA Briefing no. 21, June.

Health Development Agency (HDA) (2004b) *Taking Measures*. London: HDA, Department of Health, Liverpool John Moores University and NW Public Health Observatory. Available at: www.hda-online.org.uk (Analysis of alcohol misuse in North-West England.)

Hooper, J. and Longworth, P. (2002) *Health Needs Assessment Workbook*. London: Health Development Agency. Available at: www.hda.nhs.uk (Provides further details of health needs analysis and health impact assessment, and provides a systematic guide through the process.)

Local Government Association website: www.lga.gov.uk (Provides details of the role of local government in public health. Provides links to regional sites. Gives details of news, publications and events on a wide range of issues such as domestic violence, waste management, affordable housing and homelessness.)

National Institute for Health and Clinical Excellence (NICE) website: www.publichealth.nice.org.uk

NHS Executive (1998) *In the Public Interest: Developing a Strategy for Public Participation in the NHS*. London: Department of Health.

Phillimore, P. and Beattie, A. (1994) *Health and inequality: the northern region 1981–1991: a report*. Newcastle: University of Newcastle upon Tyne.

Quigley, R., Cavanagh, S., Hanson, D. and Taylor, L. (2003) *Clarifying Health Impact Assessment, Integrated Impact Assessment and Health Needs Assessment*. London: Health Development Agency.

Russel, H. and Killoran, A. (2000) *Public Health and Regeneration: Making the Links*. London: Health Education Authority.

Scottish Centre for Regeneration website: www.communitiesscotland.gov.uk (Provides explanation and examples of community engagement issues and participatory appraisal.)

Townsend, P., Phillimore, P. and Beattie, A. (1988) *Health and deprivation*. London: Croom Helm.

Chapter 10

Barker, W. (1990) Practical and ethical doubts about screening for child abuse, *Health Visitor*, 63(1): 14–17. (Useful reference in terms of addressing the use of screening for something other than a pathophysiological issue and also the importance and impact of sensitivity and specificity.)

DHSS (1985) *Cancer Screening (Forrest Report)*. London: HMSO. (Report of working party set up to investigate the establishment of a national breast screening programme.)

Edinburgh Well Mother website: http://www.wellmother.com/articles/edinburgh.htm (provides details of the development of the Edinburgh Postnatal Depression Score and the scoring process.)

Jepson, R., Clegg, A., Forbes, C., et al. (2000) The determinants of screening uptake and interventions for increasing uptake: a systematic review, *Health Technology Assessment*, 4(14). (This systematic review defines screening and lists a range of screening programmes.)

Last, J.M., Spasoff R.A. and Harris, S.S. (2000) *A Dictionary of Epidemiology*, 4th edn. London: International Epidemiology Association. (Classic resource for definitive definition of terms relating to epidemiology.)

National Electronic Library for Health website: www.libraries.nelh.nhs.uk/screening (Provides access to the Screening Specialist Library and to National Screening Committee's Policy Positions 2004, the latter gives details of the Committee's position on a wide range of conditions.)

NHS Cancer Screening website: www.cancerscreeening.nhs.uk (This site has links detailing incidence, screening programmes and uptake for breast, cervical, colorectal and prostate cancers.)

NHS Sickle Cell & Thalassaemia Screening Programe website: www.kcl-phs.org.uk/haem-screening (The NHS Sickle Cell and Thalassaemia Screening Programme aims to establish high quality newborn screening programmes for sickle cell disorders and antenatal screening programmes for sickle cell and thalassaemia.)

PSA Informed Choice Programme website: www.cancerscreening.nhs.uk/prostrate/index.html

Chapter 11

Adams, J. (2005) *What Kills You Matters – Not Numbers*. Available at: http://www.socialaffairsunit.org.uk/blog/archives/000512.php (The number of people killed annually in road accidents far exceeds the number killed by terrorist attacks. Yet the public fear of terrorism – and reaction to it – are on a completely different scale to that of death on the road. Prof. John Adams (Britain's leading academic expert on risk and the author of the seminal, *Risk*) asks why this should be so.)

Bennett, P. and Calman, K. (eds) (1999) *Risk Communication and Public Health*. Oxford: Oxford University Press. (This book considers public, professional and media management of risk communication. It has four sections: introduction to risk communication; review of prominent cases; institutional and political dimensions of risk communication; and exploration of key themes and practical implications.)

Connell, J. P., Kubisch, A. C., Schorr, L. B. and Weiss, C. H. (1995) *New Approaches to Evaluating Community Initiatives*. Aspen, CO: The Aspen Institute. (Considers the specific issues and characteristics of complex community initiatives.)

Pawson, R. and Tilley, N. (2004) *Realistic Evaluation*. London: Sage. (This book provides details of the context–mechanism–outcome model and provides suggestions for thinking about evaluation in different ways.)

NICE website: http://www.nice.org.uk (NICE is the independent organization responsible for providing national guidance on the promotion of good health and the prevention and treatment of ill health. On 1 April 2005 NICE joined with the Health Development Agency to become the new National Institute for Health and Clinical Excellence.)

Index

Page numbers for figures have suffix **f**, those for tables suffix **t**

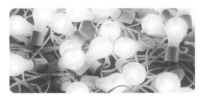 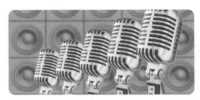
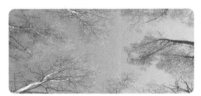 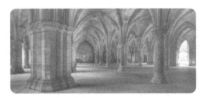
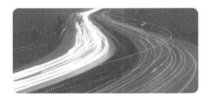 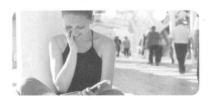
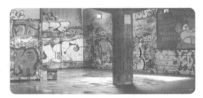